When Trauma Grips Our Children

When Trauma Grips Our Children

The Basic Pyramid System for Counselors, Teachers, and Caregivers to Support Healing

James E. Levine

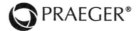 PRAEGER®

An Imprint of ABC-CLIO, LLC
Santa Barbara, California • Denver, Colorado

Library of Congress Cataloging-in-Publication Data

Names: Levine, James E., author.
Title: When trauma grips our children : the basic pyramid system for
   counselors, teachers, and caregivers to support healing / James E.
   Levine.
Description: Santa Barbara, California : Praeger, [2021] | Includes
   bibliographical references and index.
Identifiers: LCCN 2020034958 (print) | LCCN 2020034959 (ebook) | ISBN
   9781440874734 (hardcover) | ISBN 9781440874741 (ebook)
Subjects: LCSH: Psychic trauma in children—Treatment. | Post-traumatic
   stress disorder in children—Treatment. | Caregivers.
Classification: LCC RJ506.P66 L488 2021 (print) | LCC RJ506.P66 (ebook) |
   DDC 618.9285/21—dc23
LC record available at https://lccn.loc.gov/2020034958
LC ebook record available at https://lccn.loc.gov/2020034959

ISBN: 978-1-4408-7473-4 (print)
      978-1-4408-7474-1 (ebook)

25 24 23 22 21   1 2 3 4 5

This book is also available as an eBook.

Praeger
An Imprint of ABC-CLIO, LLC

ABC-CLIO, LLC
147 Castilian Drive
Santa Barbara, California 93117
www.abc-clio.com

This book is printed on acid-free paper ∞

Manufactured in the United States of America

This book discusses treatments (including types of medication and mental health therapies), diagnostic tests for various symptoms and mental health disorders, and organizations. The authors have made every effort to present accurate and up-to-date information. However, the information in this book is not intended to recommend or endorse particular treatments or organizations, or substitute for the care or medical advice of a qualified health professional, or used to alter any medical therapy without a medical doctor's advice. Specific situations may require specific therapeutic approaches not included in this book. For those reasons, we recommend that readers follow the advice of qualified health care professionals directly involved in their care. Readers who suspect they may have specific medical problems should consult a physician about any suggestions made in this book.

Contents

Acknowledgments

Writing a book like this takes more than time. The emotional investment—and sometimes, admittedly, the toll—is enormous. My deepest thanks to my wife, Cheryl Campbell, and children, Jeremy and Maya. In addition, I want to express my unending gratitude to Sophie Freud, professor emerita at Simmons University, who has been my guiding mentor in all of my writing and throughout my doctoral studies. This book would not have been possible without her input and encouragement. My thanks as well to Roger Anderson and Joanne Marqusee, who both read and commented insightfully on earlier drafts. A book like this, one that addresses deeply sensitive and challenging topics, cannot be written without such support. I am grateful to each of you.

Introduction

Children experience hellish numbers of traumatic events and conditions, including poverty, parental drug use and/or mental illness, neglect, war, dislocation, family and community strife, and physical and sexual abuse. Factor in a lack of acceptance of—and sometimes outright hostility toward—their differences in race, ethnicity, resident status, family income, religion, and sexual orientation. The list of factors that can adversely affect children is extensive and not one we should—or can—overlook. Ongoing political strife in the United States and around the world and the finger-pointing, name-calling, and endlessly polarizing commentary from those in positions of power only add to the stresses our children face. These are all magnified, of course, by social media and children's ever-present smartphones. And these factors do not even account for the typical challenges of childhood and adolescence: Who is popular, a skilled athlete, good at test taking and academics overall? As most of us recognize, childhood can be a steep uphill climb even in the best of circumstances.

Regel and Joseph (2017, p. 3) offer this simple observation: "Throughout history, it has been recognized that traumatic events can leave people in a state of confusion, distress, and despair." Fosha (2003) comments on what she calls the "unbearable aloneness" of living with trauma. This book explains how trauma contributes to that sense of loneliness and shows some of what we can do when a child is hurting and needs our help.

When a child is living with trauma, what does it look like? There is no single picture, but we often see children who, on the one hand, rage at the world, even at those people who may be trying to help them. As one woman told me in reflecting on her childhood, she exuded anger through her pores. She hit, spit, ran away, and hid. These children may become agitated over the smallest challenges and disagreements, exploding over what may appear to be an insignificant problem. They are often described as edgy, controlling, and defiant. On the other hand, we see children who shut down and seem disengaged, even vacant. They may avoid others and stay as far in the background as they can. For many such children, the word *anxious* (and sometimes *panicky*) is applied. In both of these scenarios, we often experience them as mistrusting, inattentive, and even erratic. I hear these various descriptions used on a daily basis.

It has become virtually a social movement to talk about this word *trauma*. A term formerly reserved for military personnel and first responders such as firefighters and police officers, it seems that now almost everyone, including our children, can be described as having survived trauma. The diagnosis of PTSD, or post-traumatic stress disorder, was not formally introduced into the psychological literature until 1980, which means that the idea of addressing trauma as a recognized mental health concern is relatively new. Clearly, not everyone is in distress, yet the word has evolved as an entrenched aspect of our cultural language and discussion. We have work to do to better describe what we mean and, even more so, to explain how we intend to act when we encounter children experiencing profound suffering. Otherwise we run the risk of accepting trauma as just "something that happens." Although Lifton (2017) used this chilling phrase in a different context, it applies here and now as well: *malignant normality*. We do not want childhood suffering to become something we accept or tolerate as the natural state of things.

Another term we commonly hear is *safety*. Children need to feel safe, and *psychological safety* is all the rage. How do we nurture it, especially among children whose life experiences have taught that they may have good reason to feel unsafe?

School counselors, teachers, administrators, parents, and other caregivers— this book is for you—tell me that many of these terms are used so loosely as to have lost all practical meaning. This does not negate their significance but only their capacity to be translated into practice. The goal of promoting— never mind teaching—safety and resilience causes middle-of-the-night apprehension and, in the sage words of one counselor, leads to an empty, frustrating search down a maze of dark alleyways. Yes, we now have a burgeoning marketplace of expensive social-emotional learning (SEL) programs, but these do not necessarily reach all children, especially those with deep-seated emotional and behavioral problems linked to trauma. Ask any teacher if the classroom's SEL curriculum is effective for the teacher's most angry, defiant, or shut-down students, and it is not hard to anticipate the answer. Across the board, I am told that it does not lead to any kind of consistent success with this group of children.

The point of this book is not to pathologize traumatized children. The point is to understand their struggle and develop meaningful ways to help them. While some of the *what's wrong* will be discussed, so, too, will post-traumatic growth, resilience, and the *what works*.

If we are going to talk about making schools and homes safe for children, let's design a trauma-informed framework for *how* to do so. Physical safety is an obvious goal, but how do teachers and caregivers create and maintain psychological safety, especially for children who have experienced severe forms of trauma? As a young clinician, I had no real clue how to proceed toward this laudable objective. That dark maze of alleyways is a place I stumbled a fair amount of time while searching for a better understanding and some useful strategies. We have made progress on the former; there has been almost a kind of consciousness-raising around the subject of trauma. But I am not sure that the latter has grown in any structured, coherent way beyond the walls of therapists' offices. An exception is Jennings's (2019) addition to the literature, which provides an overview of trauma in the school setting. In a broader way, Ablon's (2018) work on a model he calls Collaborative Problem Solving describes helpful ways to bring a different approach to discipline and, overall, to think about children's negative behaviors from a *skills deficit* perspective rather than a willful one. My hope is to shed additional light on the subject and to offer new ideas for intervention.

To achieve this, each chapter is geared to the larger goal of broadening the discussion around trauma, primarily in school settings, but in ways that can also be applied by a parent or other caregivers. Chapter 1 defines some of the important terms and concepts that underlie psychological safety through an exploration of childhood trauma and related concerns. We will also look at the seminal Adverse Childhood Experiences study, behaviors related to trauma, and the subtle distinction between the *functions* and *meaning* of children's behavior. Chapter 2 offers a framework for creating safety (or what I will call "support") plans, primarily in school settings but that can also be adapted by caregivers to use at home. I refer to this model of support planning as "the Basic Pyramid," usually shortened simply to "the Pyramid." Chapter 3 explores the differences between these interventions and formal behavioral plans. Additionally, it addresses ideas for how to talk with children about using a support plan, something that does not come easily to many of us. Chapters 4 and 5 delve into the important topics of shame and lying and describe why children with trauma sometimes exhibit their own unique quality to how and when they lie. When they do so, they are at greater risk of additional stress, depression, punishment by others, and social isolation. Chapter 6 addresses the critical idea of "restitution," more commonly referred to as "restorative practice" or "restorative justice." Restitution is a primary way to help children reduce the shame they carry. In addition, this chapter shows how restitution is based on teaching children the skills they need so that they can understand the impact of their behavior on others. Chapter 7 looks at diagnoses that commonly occur in conjunction with post-traumatic stress disorder (PTSD) as well as the topic of children's meaning making. Chapter 8 describes elements of psychotherapy for children with trauma, how to adapt them to nonclinical settings, and ways they can be integrated into the Pyramid. In addition, we will look at the notions of resilience and post-traumatic growth. Chapter 9 applies the model and these ideas to two children, Esther and Jake (not their real names), who are struggling in school. The final chapter offers concluding thoughts, directions, and questions for the future.

A note: Stories you may find painful to read and think about are included in this book. They are a kind of witnessing for every reader. Trauma entails some of the worst of humanity, and the case studies and comments reflect exactly that. Knowing that children experience disturbing, even cruel, acts is likely not a surprise to anyone, but hearing about them in some detail, as well as trying to digest children's own words, is altogether different. These are all based on true stories, carefully disguised in composite form to protect children's privacy. Please know that we will also discuss post-traumatic *growth*, the notion that children can and do overcome severe circumstances and ultimately thrive. That, of course, is the goal we hold for every traumatized child.

This book was primarily written before the 2020 advent of the coronavirus and its dramatic impact on all our lives. COVID-19 has not done away with trauma; if anything, trauma has increased for vast numbers of children and their families. Illness, job loss, isolation, and the sudden disappearance of predictability, structure, and a fundamental sense of normalcy have changed our understanding and experience of the world. For so many, there is less feeling of safety than there was before.

One bright spot, which I have observed through many ongoing (remote) discussions with counselors and principals, is a newfound sense of the benefits—and joys—of working collaboratively. While before, there was often a sense of "not enough time," the new order has brought about a blossoming of a team approach that I never witnessed before, at least not to this extent. Using the Pyramid, and thinking deeply about specific children who struggle the most, will not seem so out of place in our new way of doing things, that is, if we choose to continue practicing some of these new ways.

The virus, in its insidious way, magnifies what works and what doesn't in children's lives. Let's all make sure we address their needs in the ways they require of us. At the same time, we must also take care of ourselves and our own networks of family, friends, and community during these unsettled days.

CHAPTER ONE

Trauma and Psychological Safety

Children need to feel safe. We understand this implicitly, but ask almost anyone who spends a significant chunk of time with them to clearly define the term *safety*. And beyond that, ask them to outline the elements of what creates safety. These have always been complex and intriguing questions for me. Maybe the best way to start is a simple approach: Ask children to define what it means for them. If needed, I will float some possible descriptions of safety if the children cannot come up with any on their own. This can be a delicate process depending on how guarded or defended the individual children are, and it is one among many ways in which we confront the complications of a given child's trauma.

If we are going to talk about creating safety, we need to look first at what it means for a child to live with trauma. The literature on childhood trauma is broad. And it is abundant: Some describe *what* trauma is, some define the characteristics of children's emotional and behavioral responses, and some offer general rules of thumb on how to help. In the psychotherapy literature, there is ample discussion of different interventions that can be effective for those children fortunate enough to access a skilled trauma therapist. What we do not have is a sturdy enough framework for the daily or even moment-to-moment decisions that underlie what we actually *do*, especially when we are faced with an angry, sometimes seething or, conversely, a shut-down and inaccessible child.

We rarely hear the words of children describing their own experiences or, for that matter, the voices of teachers trying to balance rigorous classroom learning with an empathic response to distressed students. Nor, frankly, do we often hear from counselors about the stories they sit with every day. In my supervision sessions, counselors commonly share stories of children who hurt themselves, who lash out at others, who cannot concentrate on school because they are distracted from the here-and-now of trying to make sense of their lives, or who struggle to understand relationships and others' intentions. In short, they are angry, confused, anxious, and discouraged. As painful as they are to witness, all of these stories are fertile sources for understanding trauma at a deeper level.

The best definitions of trauma emphasize the individual's response to a heightened situation. One perspective is that it is "a psychologically distressing event that is outside the range of usual human experience, often involving a sense of intense fear, terror, and helplessness" (Perry, 2007, p. 15). To me, this is, to borrow from the world of scientific research, a necessary but not sufficient description. A better one is this: "Trauma is defined by its effect on a particular individual's nervous system, *not on the intensity* of the circumstance itself" (Levine & Kline, 2006, p. 5). Ten children may witness the same frightening event; most will not be affected in any significant, long-term way while others, maybe one or two or perhaps three, may develop full-blown post-traumatic stress disorder, or PTSD. There is a host of factors that contribute to the outcome, including a child's temperament, social supports, prior history, and the degree of parents' mental health.

Fisher (2017), whose work focuses primarily on adults with trauma, offers two powerful words of description: *self-alienation* and *fragmentation*. Her terms imply the consequences of severe trauma, the idea of feeling "less than whole," a phrase used by an adolescent I worked with in therapy, and the experience of being both distant from and unable to make sense of those fragmented pieces of oneself. Davies (2018, p. 114) offers another succinct definition, referring to trauma as the "psychological pattern of seeking control over suffering."

According to the website of the National Child Traumatic Stress Network (2019), there are three main types of trauma: acute, chronic, and complex.

- Acute trauma results from a single incident.
- Chronic trauma is repeated and prolonged such as domestic violence or abuse.
- Complex trauma is exposure to varied and multiple traumatic events, often of an invasive, interpersonal nature.

The acronym TRAINCRASH (Saxe et al., 1993) is a comprehensive way to describe and remember the characteristic elements of trauma, as follows:

1. Core symptoms
    -Traumatic experiencing
    -Reexperiencing

　　　-Avoidance

　　　-Increased arousal

　　　-Numbing

2.　Associated features

　　　-Conscious alterations (dissociation)

　　　-Relationship difficulties

　　　-Affect dysregulation

　　　-Somatization of symptoms

　　　-Harmful behavior

Perhaps a plainer way to characterize these elements is to say that trauma affects virtually every aspect of children's lives: how they feel physically and emotionally; how they experience their environment; how they think (and what enters their conscious minds); and how they treat others and, maybe even more so, themselves. Using these different criteria, it is not difficult to conceptualize the challenges that arise.

Among very young children, you can see a startling lack of symbolic play. Sorrels (2015), an early childhood specialist, describes children who are concrete in their thinking to the point that they cannot engage in pretend play. She shares an example of a three-year-old who was unable to talk on an imaginary telephone; he could not make sense of the object, even though he understood what a telephone was, and threw it on the floor. She observed the same with a five-year-old who, at least at first, could not engage in this kind of play. When he made sense of it, she reports, he smiled with delight. These examples point to the developmental lags that can occur as a result of abuse.

Another outcome of trauma is that praise can be uniquely difficult for traumatized children. For those who live with chronic trauma, compliments are not necessarily something to celebrate; they can be followed by a swift reversal and terrible outcomes. And, for many, their self-understanding can be made so negative that approval of any kind is not only dismissed but also causes literal discomfort and stress. The following quote, from an author who grew up in a family beset by severe bipolar disorder and possible psychosis, reflects this perfectly—and painfully: "I could tolerate any form of cruelty better than kindness. Praise was a poison to me; I choked on it" (Westover, 2018, p. 240).

As noted, if we use the preceding criteria, they reveal that trauma is not the disturbing event itself; it is a child's internal response to that event. There are behavioral guidelines to help us determine if a child suffers from trauma. Like any diagnosis, and like any human condition, there is a continuum. I have spoken with both children and adults mildly affected by a horrific event or history, and I have sat with others who are devastated by comparable experiences. There are similarities in how they react, if not in degree but in type, including thoughts that intrude at unexpected times, sleep problems, nightmares, a perception of things being threatening and out of control, and a general sense of edginess, unease, and mistrust. We see these symptoms, although they may present differently, in all age groups.

Information reported by Stanford Children's Health (2019) and published on their website supports these same symptoms of PTSD during childhood. They also note high rates of anxiety and depression and a greater risk of substance abuse. Physical symptoms like stomachaches and headaches are common, as is irritability. Stanford researchers also refer to "reenactment" of a traumatic event, something we often see in a child's behavior or even in his play. There is, frankly, ample literature describing the perils of living with trauma.

A study out of Penn State University (Jones, Lam, Hoffer, Chen, & Schreier, 2018) found that adolescents who live with "chronic family stress" have a higher risk of persistent health problems as they grow into adulthood. Depending on the type of coping skills they use—"cognitive reappraisal" versus "suppression"—their outcomes will vary. This gives us an important rationale for focusing on teaching coping skills, especially for children with trauma. On the surface, trying to suppress negative thoughts may seem helpful—just ignore them and keep going—but these researchers found it advantageous for this group of adolescents to learn how to reframe their stress in a more positive way, that is, from a different perspective than they held previously, especially one that does not contribute to their often excessive self-blame.

The Adverse Childhood Experiences (ACEs) Study

By now, many educators and counselors are familiar with the Adverse Childhood Experiences (ACEs) study. A seminal investigation conducted many years ago, it was, and remains today, instrumental in showing that living with various forms of stress is closely related to emotional and body-based struggles. Conducted between 1995 and 1997 through a joint effort by the Centers for Disease Control and Prevention and Kaiser Permanente, the study addressed factors such as family separation and substance abuse, poverty, a family history of mental illness, domestic violence in the home, and physical and sexual abuse—in other words, various forms of toxic stress. Unlike previous, small-scale studies, this one employed a huge number of participants, more than 17,000 in all.

Among many important findings, what emerged from the study is that as children experience an increasing number of adverse childhood experiences, they are significantly more likely to face a host of behavioral health and medical problems. Even though the study was conducted more than 20 years ago, its findings are still relevant today. It makes implicit sense that the greater the stress, the more likely one is to struggle in various ways. This study, however, provides strong empirical support for what we could only assume we knew.

Knowing about these findings, and therefore the risks to children's well-being, makes the reality of this country's documented rise in opioid abuse even more shocking. It is rarely just an "individual" event; an overdose, whether it leads to detox, rehabilitation, incarceration, or even death, very often affects a child. It impacts a son, a daughter, a relative, or a family friend. I rarely visit a school where this is not a reality for one or more children. The ACEs study helps us to comprehend why so many of them are struggling.

The potential dangers of childhood, and the countless stories molded by those experiences, are in many ways reflected in the specific questions posed to participants in the study. While the richness of children's narratives is not something we get to see and experience directly, the ACEs investigation provides data that are nonetheless illuminating. Never before did we have concrete information that showed us, throughout our entire life span, how much children's toxic experiences could hinder them. It revealed that, without help, support, and some effective interventions, a child could struggle developmentally across virtually *all* aspects of growing up.

We can look at this from an *ecological* perspective. In short, ecological theory is "fundamentally concerned with the interaction and interdependence of organisms and their environment. . . . Individuals, families, groups and communities interact with their environments and are shaped by them" (Teater, 2014, p. 36). As such, there is an entwined relationship among a child's experience of the world, the nature and depth of the child's significant relationships, and the child's genetic makeup. In the mental health fields, there is a similar emphasis on what is called the *biopsychosocial* approach. In short, it integrates the view of a child's biology, psychological factors, and social relationships to understand health and wellness or, as is common among children with trauma histories, the lack of them.

The ACEs study gives us needed data for understanding that trauma increases health risks across all areas. Trauma, we know, starts as an outside-in event. Something *happens* to a child, whether directly or as witness, and the child *reacts*—physically, emotionally, socially, behaviorally, and even spiritually. Trauma, therefore, is experiential. Yet it is the collision of that experience with the child's inborn traits and style of relating—the child's temperament, as well as history and level of social support—that determines whether the child will develop the formal signs of PTSD. Any parent with more than one child knows that children are born with widely varying traits. I have seen parents marvel at how one child may be shy, even withdrawn, when the other is outgoing and continually searching for social connections. In 1977, psychiatrists Thomas and Chess identified three basic types or "clusters" of temperament: easy, difficult, and slow to warm up. It seems obvious that children in the first group, who tend to be tranquil, see things more positively and adapt more easily to new situations; they have the best odds for facing a traumatic event and coming through it without a long-term negative impact. An ecological view allows us to see children in the fullness of their life experience and temperamental style—the combination of such factors—rather than as merely the passive recipients of what life throws at them.

Behaviors

Children formally diagnosed with PTSD demonstrate a broad range of behaviors. They are, of course, much more than their diagnosis, a notion that at times gets lost when people hear the word *trauma*. (I see this same kind of narrow lens when the term *autism* is voiced.) That is, we may make rigid assumptions about a child based solely on a diagnostic term. Instead, we should recall that behavior serves as a primary way to communicate (Levine, 2007), and this is especially true for children who may not have the words to label their experiences or their emotions. If it were only that simple and children could reliably describe their internal states, psychotherapy—not to mention parenting and teaching—would be easier and more straightforward. Our sometimes sleepless nights as adults reflect that the process of helping such children is anything but easy and straightforward. It speaks to children's complexity and the wide spectrum of behaviors they display beyond the mere fact of a trauma designation.

Children, especially those who do not receive help, tend to divide into one of two distinct groups when they have experienced trauma. There are the *externalizers*, those who act out their pain for the world to see. They may be highly depressed, but the depression is revealed like a shot out of a cannon. They are typically argumentative, often disruptive, and sometimes strongly oppositional if not aggressive. Caregivers, teachers, and administrators complain about these children, because it is difficult to reason with them. They do not necessarily or consistently respond to consequences, whether negative or positive, because the capacity to think logically and in sequence (if I do A, then B will happen) can be weakened as a result of their trauma. This is not a statement about a child's intelligence or character; rather, it speaks to how any of us can have the calm, rational aspects of our brain captured by anxiety, powerful emotions, and the sense that we are spiraling out of control. This is why formal behavioral plans often do not work for these children: When they do not earn the reward they anticipate, they often end up angry or rageful, clearly not the outcome we want, and unable to process the ensuing feedback. In other words, the behavioral interventions do not work as *teaching* tools, their primary reason for being. And it is the same reason why ultimatums, threats, and mention of major consequences usually backfire. Typically, these will not change behavior for the better, but we may well end up instead with a fuming, even aggressive, child in front of us, one who is overwhelmed, dysregulated, feeling threatened, and even less able to regain control.

Internalizers shift in the opposite direction. When under stress, they may end up in full shut-down mode, where verbal dialogue is impossible. Children who cope in this way (similar to adults with trauma) describe such a state as unpleasant, frightening, and unintentional, even though they may be accused of doing it on purpose. I hear this complaint regularly, that the child is being "willful." Some children describe this experience as having been "taken over" by a feeling of flatness and the inability to mobilize their own resources, whether it is a matter of problem-solving, logical thinking, or even the use of language. Mental processing, or *processing speed*, has been shown to slow down during these times as well, making it even more challenging to manage. In extreme scenarios, people can become catatonic, unable to organize themselves enough to move their bodies in a purposeful way.

We know this kind of withdrawal as *dissociation*. It is a clinical term that many people, professionals and nonprofessionals alike, recognize. How it shows up in children with PTSD, however, is less well recognized. For example, some children will smirk when in this state, and it appears to an observer that they are purposely aiming to get attention from an adult. But if you were to inspect the child's *eyes* rather than the slight upturn at the corner of the child's lips, you would see what appears to be a blank or vacant look. I have interviewed children and adults alike who reported either no or very dim memory of that time, suggesting the facial expression was anything but an attempt to be noticed. The default assumption, however, is that the child is being rebellious and attention-seeking. It can certainly appear that way in the moment when the child is not doing what is asked and displays what presents as (and, to us, often feels like) a look of pure defiance. In the most acute crisis situations, I have seen children smear their own blood or feces without having any recollection afterward.

A confounding aspect of trauma, one that prompts confusion and no small amount of concern, is that children with PTSD can become distracted and upset not by a specific event that occurs in their immediate environment but by a *thought* or visual image that suddenly and without warning intrudes into their conscious awareness. We see similar episodes in people with schizophrenia. This is known as *internal stimuli*, the opposite of what we usually search for when a child gets triggered. Mandler (2012) refers to them more generally as "mind-pops," suggesting that they can occur during any activity, including the most routine ones. Even in a relatively controlled environment where things may not have changed in any significant way, a calm, focused child can suddenly become upset, distracted, volatile, or withdrawn. Keeping in mind the idea of an ecological approach to understanding trauma, it recognizes that one's recall of a negative experience can be driven by unexpected stimuli and unforeseen moments, not just specific external events. It also raises again the question of how we can help a child feel protected. As one girl poignantly told me, "If my thoughts aren't okay, I have nowhere to go to be safe. I can't hide in my bed from those."

Research regarding adolescents with depression, although I would argue that this is equally if not even more relevant for those with PTSD, outlines what it calls *negative emotion differentiation* (NED). The investigators (Starr, Hershenberg, Shaw, Li, & Santee, 2019) define NED in terms of how effectively a child is able to identify and label specific negative emotions. In depressed adolescents, they found that this group of children is significantly less skilled than others of the same age. They further suggested that, as a result, lower NED is associated with a higher degree of depression, especially when *stressful life events* (SLEs) are present. If you cannot identify your emotions or put a specific name to them during high-pressure moments, they become bigger, more frightening, and increasingly overwhelming. By extension, this would inevitably contribute to further externalizing or internalizing behavior as a result.

Another hallmark of PTSD is *regression*, essentially the idea that someone can suddenly begin to function at a lower developmental level. They become younger and less mature in their behavior and speech, especially when under stress. Seeing it in action can be dramatic. In an emergency room setting, I witnessed a man who, in conversation with me, went from acting like an approximately 30-year-old adult to a screaming, thrashing toddler having a full-blown temper tantrum. This included stomping his feet, making faces, and behaving like a three-year-old during an overexhausted meltdown. All of us have the capacity to regress to some degree, but it is unusual to see someone backslide to such an extent. It spoke to the depth of this man's trauma and, at that moment, his inability to manage it. Some people in the waiting room watched and gaped, others found it somewhat amusing, but I felt sad for him. While this may seem a rather extreme example, it is anything but unique. It is regression in raw form.

In another example of regression that teachers report on a fairly frequent basis, some children with trauma will put themselves under a desk in school when they get frustrated with a task or become upset in general. We see something similar in particular children with autism, which is often due to their need to shut down sensory stimuli. (At times, children on the spectrum will hide in cubbies, lockers, or classroom closets. They have the same underlying reason: to reduce overstimulation.) For traumatized children, there certainly may be a sensory aspect to this behavior as well—to cut down on light, sound, and the eye gaze of others—and it may also be due to needing to avoid a task or an interaction. As we will discuss, avoidance is central to trauma, but it can represent regression as well. Some children who at other times may be able to talk about what is going on for them and make reasoned decisions will go under a desk when they are overwhelmed and unable to manage. Often, this is viewed as purposeful, acting-out behavior, but a trauma-informed perspective suggests otherwise: that it relates to a direct inability to cope in the moment. One 5th-grade boy practically spit out the words when he told me, "I know I look stupid, and that the other kids think it's weird. I can't help it. Why do I always get in trouble for it?"

Other regressive behaviors we see in traumatized children include whining, yelling, baby-talk, and even thumb-sucking. Some children suddenly become clingy with adults. While these are most certainly disruptive in a classroom setting, they should be addressed as a form of regression—which means we focus on trying to calm the child—rather than as purposeful and intentional. To clarify, I am not at all suggesting that children do not ever purposefully act out, but in this context, the behaviors represent something else. And strategically, you will see that emphasizing calming rather than discipline when this occurs will lead to a better outcome.

Boundaries: A simple definition of boundaries is this: They are "guidelines, rules, or limits that a person creates to identify reasonable, safe and permissible ways for other people to behave towards them and how they will respond when someone passes those limits" (Richmond, 2018). Learning about and maintaining good boundaries is a developmental challenge for every child, and it is magnified many times over for children with trauma. As one reflective, self-aware adolescent told me, "I've been violated a hundred times. How the hell would I know anything about how to read other people or even be with them? I don't know if I'm getting too close, too far; I have no way to tell." This rings true in the comments offered by so many children who have been abused, especially if it was by those they trusted. In a sense, their boundaries were obliterated, and this reveals itself through how difficult it is for them to then maintain a reasonable, safe distance from others. I have witnessed children who will clamor to sit on your lap or hug you tightly, even if you are a complete stranger to them, and children who will gravitate to a far corner and go to great lengths to rebuff any attempt to engage them. Forming a sense of how to be comfortable relating to other people—or even tolerate being in their presence—is not an automatic skill, and we commonly see this struggle in children who have not been taught or modeled healthy ways to interact with others.

Predictability: In my work in schools, what is notable is the extent to which children with trauma seek predictability and consistency. As a group, they need to know what to expect, when things will happen, and who will be there. And, to a significant degree, they need to know that they will not fail. Making mistakes may be a learning opportunity—and we remind children of this all the time—but for these children, mistakes may have led to serious and even dangerous outcomes. One adolescent reported that if he dropped something at home—a dish, a cup, his shoes a little too loudly on the floor—his mother's boyfriend would gesture wildly, threaten, and on occasion hit him. There was no way to predict which response would come. Later, his concerns about making any kind of mistake in school, even though he understood intellectually that he would not be hurt by anyone there, led to profound worry and a relentless, unsatisfying drive to be "perfect."

If we understand trauma partially as one's experience of having lost control—over one's body, one's safety, one's ability to make coherent sense of the world—it seems evident that the ability to anticipate events could provide at least a temporary sense of control. In short, one knows what to expect. Children with trauma often gravitate to anything that allows them to regain this sense, even if temporarily, but it comes at a steep price. Perfectionism and unyielding anxiety are the cost; and rigidity—"I don't want anything to change; nothing *can* change, or I won't be able to handle it"—is another.

Fear of change and the need for control: To live with these kinds of internal restrictions, according to one young adult, is to confine one's life to the point of near absurdity. It is no wonder that many children with trauma, especially when it is yet to be revealed, start with diagnoses like anxiety, depression, and obsessive-compulsive disorder. Each diagnosis lends itself to a pressing sense of powerlessness. Some children with trauma are not identified until they have made active attempts at suicide. One adolescent told me point-blank after his second attempt that he felt helpless, hopeless, and worthless, a classic triad representing high suicide risk. The attempt to end his life was, in his words, the only way he could take control of a situation that felt beyond his ability to cope.

This perception of lacking any control over one's life mounts a serious obstacle to developing a healthy identity, the primary development task of adolescence. It may also affect a child's expectation for some degree of consistency, or even a basic level of fairness, from caregivers. And because so many children with trauma make desperate attempts to take control of their environments, they may inadvertently push away other children, damaging the possibility for maintaining friendships. They can frustrate their teachers, counselors, and caregivers with the incessant need to be in charge such that they come to be viewed as oppositional and defiant. This need to take control—if we could step into their shoes, we would see—is a survival tactic, not intentional behavior, but we typically receive it as purposeful and aimed at pushing our buttons. Adults with their own high need for control can find this behavior especially intolerable. As one 7th-grade teacher (who acknowledged her own challenging history) candidly told me, she and her student with PTSD were a "match made in hell." Neither one knew how to step back rather than jump right into the fray; major power struggles were the inevitable result.

Trust: It seems obvious that a history of severe trauma, especially if it involves sexual or physical violence, will contribute to a deepening sense—a belief system, as one child told me—that others cannot be trusted. As that same child told me sadly, "I don't trust the idea of trust." Even the concept itself was fraught with pain and confusion. Less apparent, however, is what happens afterward in relationships when a child does not or cannot trust. When I began to explore this question more closely, a consistent observation emerged; primarily, it revolves around a getting-close-and-pulling-away dynamic. Most counselors and teachers have experienced this without necessarily attaching such a relational and behavioral pattern to trauma: A child feels connected and shares personal moments and stories, whether serious or lighthearted, but the next day—or sometimes, later the same day if not immediately afterward—the child is angry, sullen, or withdrawn. The interaction takes on a different tone. So what happened?

One 14-year-old girl, Tasha, expressed that the feeling of connection, or, maybe a better term, *connectedness*, leads to a bitter sense of fear and dread. She had felt close to someone who, after long sessions of drinking, broke her trust so brutally and unpredictably that she came to believe that connectedness, the fundamental sense of a meaningful attachment, could only be linked to a wrenching betrayal. Given this, whenever she began to get close to someone at school—a teacher, a counselor, even other students—the only option available to her was to pull away. This was not done gently. Usually, it took the form of anger, blame, and, internally, a crushing sense of shame, since she recognized that others weren't necessarily out to hurt her. Her intellectual brain knew this, but her emotional brain could not hold the idea. She described the experience as being "overtaken" with strong emotions that "seem to make the decisions for me." Volcanic rages were sometimes the result. Tasha broke a lot of chairs at school and various items at home.

As a young clinician, I worked with a 12-year-old boy, Kevin, whose life up until the year before, when he was finally removed from his house and placed in a foster home, could only be described as hell on earth. He lived in filth with virtually no adult attention or oversight; the word *neglect* does not begin to describe it. His mother had subjected him to terrible, humiliating acts. Slowly, over time, this boy and I developed a meaningful relationship, and, frankly, I enjoyed his company. As wounded as he was in some ways, he was also deeply interested in nature and in being outdoors. There were kernels of real joy for him in these activities, and I saw his kind, warm side when he talked about animals. Often we took walks when we met, since this was more comfortable for him. (At one point he joked about being like a "caged animal" when he had to sit in an office or classroom.) As I began to believe he was starting to trust me, he came in one day with fire in his eyes and told me in no uncertain terms that he "hated" me and then would not talk or move for the rest of the session. I have never forgotten those moments, which for me were filled with confusion, worry, and deep sadness. It was only later that I came to understand that he feared the trust we were developing. The nice news is that we were able to move past it; I receive a holiday card from this now grown man every year.

Another example is that of Ron, who was 15 and one very angry boy. His trauma history consisted of a drug-abusing stepfather and physical abuse by his birth father, who was no longer in his life. Ron was the kind of kid whose look could pierce right through you; he was the epitome of controlled rage waiting to be unleashed. Sometimes, when we sat in the same room, I would suddenly and without warning visualize a cobra. Like Kevin, he preferred walking to sitting, but only after we had spent enough time in my office for him, I believe, to trust that I would not abandon or hurt him outside that space. We took to walking at almost every session, and there were times I could describe as almost pleasant. He was less guarded and more talkative while we marched in a long loop that took us by a small, well-kept memorial park. Like much of New England, this little place blossomed fully in May— flowering trees, bulbs springing up everywhere—and it was beautiful and peaceful all at once. One day that month, Ron asked me if I brought other kids to this same park, and after a moment's consideration as to whether I should first ask why he wanted to know, I said no. I told him I walked there myself at times and occasionally with other clinicians from the clinic, but he was the only child I had been there with.

In my mind, I was emphasizing to Ron that he was special to me; he had significance beyond being "just another client." He seemed genuinely to appreciate this, at least if his facial expression was an accurate measure. But for the next few weeks, he was adamant that he would not leave the building with me; he was angry, sarcastic—"dripping" with sarcasm comes to mind— and uncommunicative. Finally, the light bulb went off in my head, much later than I would have wished: It probably scared Ron to no end to be seen as special, an experience foreign to him, especially with adult men, and he wondered when he would then be viewed as unspecial. In other words, he was waiting for me to abandon him. He did not—or could not at that time— trust our relationship. I proposed this idea to him—carefully, in real talk rather than therapist-speak—and he dismissed it instantly, and with a memorable sneer still grafted into my visual memory. But, interestingly, we went back to taking walks the very next session. Our relationship had its ups and downs when he perceived he had revealed too much of himself or that he was getting too close to me (or me to him), but he began to figure out how to tell me in words rather than shut down or avoid showing up for his appointment. This was a new skill for him, one built on a more than two-year relationship with a clinician that he tentatively, with many painful fits and starts, began to trust.

Brown (2015) comments on what he describes as the "opposite" of trust. He suggests that, cognitively, it is represented by *doubt*. Adults can be astonished by how even the simplest, most straightforward statements are met with skepticism. While this is often interpreted as defiance, it can be linked to a child's history of trauma. A teacher reported that no matter what he said in the classroom, one student—Jonny, a boy with a lengthy history of trauma (and no intellectual or learning deficits)—looked at him quizzically, even when straight facts were presented. It was as though Jonny disbelieved or was puzzled by virtually everything that came out of his teacher's mouth, particularly when it was something he had not heard before. Fortunately, his teacher did not perceive the boy's facial expression as oppositional, but he struggled with how to make sense of it. Using a trauma-informed perspective helped him not only with his understanding but also with how he then worked to develop a more personal relationship with Jonny. This boy had put up such a wall that it was easy to assume he wanted everyone to stay away, which was not at all the story. It was a choppy progression and took a while before Jonny was able to listen to his teacher in the classroom without assuming some hidden, negative message. Opening himself up to someone else was intimidating but, gradually, it happened.

Doubt may be a thinking-level response to trauma but, according to Brown, *fear* is the emotional reaction. This is a critical distinction. Kevin was a living example. He could lash out wildly when he was not sure about someone's motives. Our 14-year-old, Tasha, articulated this perfectly. She reported that life was like "living in a horror movie" in terms of her ongoing level of dread. Describing herself as "overwhelmed" with what one traumatized adult aptly termed "giant emotions" is similar to what we hear from people of all ages with PTSD. It tells us that such a response, while it may be unproductive in so many situations, is easy to comprehend in this context. When it is a matter of a single individual, we are likely to look at and possibly blame the individual for the individual's actions; when it happens consistently among so many different people with PTSD, we should realize that it says something about the commonality of how they internalize their experience. This, of course, is exactly what an ecological or biopsychosocial view would suggest. But it is not easy to adopt such an intellectual understanding when someone is sprinting away in full-blown flight mode, uttering vicious statements, snarling, or shutting down in front of our eyes.

If we accept Brown's observation that fear is the primary emotional response to a lack of trust, we can better understand the implications. Fear underlies the state of *fight, flight, or freeze*. While it makes sense in theory, it is harder to remember in practice. For adults, when a child shuts down and will not respond, acknowledge us, or even move, our own anxiety or anger can kick in, exacerbating the stress already present in the room. Or if that child acts unexpectedly, whether through sudden verbal defiance or aggressive behavior, it takes mental and emotional effort to step back and hold on to its fundamental cause. Not everyone deals effectively with heightened individuals, especially when logic, reason, or genuine kindness may not work in the moment. Trust, therefore, is a vastly more complex phenomenon than we might anticipate or even recognize.

Attachment is also a much-discussed concept. We know, according to Ainsworth's groundbreaking research published in 1978, that there are three distinct types or styles. She identifies (1) secure (type B), (2) insecure avoidant (type A), and (3) insecure ambivalent/resistant (type C). My 14-year-old client, Tasha, fell into the third category, wanting and then not wanting connection. Clearly, and for good reason, children with abuse histories struggle to develop secure attachment. It is possible to conceptualize this lack of trust as a coping skill rather than some sort of deficit, at least within the confines of the abusive relationship. The inability to step out of this kind of coping, to distinguish when a relationship is safe enough to alter one's attachment style, is what leads to high levels of uncertainty and distress. It also contributes directly to isolation and the experience of "unbearable aloneness."

Maggie, a nine-year-old who has already lived in many different short-term foster homes, seems almost constantly to be in transition. She cycles in and out of her father's home and back into foster care, which contributes to a child who, upon meeting her, might best be described as a whirlwind of motion and activity. Funny, smart, easy to laugh, she is also filled with anxiety and strikes me as a living portrayal of insecure attachment (type C). Given her history, this is anything but surprising; she can predict and depend on very little. One of the primary struggles her school faces is that, during those periods when she lives with her father, she often misses stretches of school days or arrives late. When she does come in, there is a massive struggle in the parking lot to get her into the building. This is not an unfamiliar scenario for many school counselors and administrators when interacting with school-phobic or school-avoidant children, but it is a time-consuming and emotional process for everyone involved. Maggie is in complete fight-or-flight mode at these times, at least until she can transition into the counselor's office and de-escalate. Afterward, she seems sad and downcast. The school is, to say the least, concerned, but staff understand why this occurs and demonstrate an admirable level of patience. It is clear that they care deeply about this girl. Her insecure attachment with her father manifests not merely in contained anger or anxiety but in total panic. Solms (2019) predicts exactly this state when a severe form of insecure attachment is in force, suggesting that it is followed by grief. As such, we should not be shocked when this kind of reactivity surfaces.

Insecure attachment is traditionally viewed as a temperament style, a *trait* rather than a changeable *state*. Yet I have seen children scarred by trauma who, with the right supports, can alter the fundamental nature of how they enter and maintain trusting relationships. It is a tentative, back-and-forth development that, when successful, unfolds over time and leads to less upheaval in their significant relationships. Current neuroscientific research (see Siegel, 2012) points repeatedly to how these changes, while they may coincide with strong emotions and relationship challenges during the process, lead to *physical* changes in the architecture of a child's brain as they form more stable relationships.

So, what does insecure attachment, or leaky trust—one child was highly amused when I referred to it in this way, especially because she loved boats—mean for the adult-student relationship in school? Often it means that the adult needs to accept that this relational coming and going is central to childhood trauma. I have witnessed teachers and counselors become sad, deeply hurt, and even outwardly angry because they perceive that the relationship has broken down; they may then blame the child—or blame themselves—and pull away, an undeniably human reaction but one that will lead to greater stress for the child and likely reinforce the child's belief that adults cannot be trusted. Knowing that the anger, the withdrawal, and the pulling away in all its different forms are most likely intermittent and a way for the child to maintain a sense of safety allows us to stay present and curious rather than angry or anxious. It means we do not pull away from her, but we do not pursue her either. We are there when she is ready to take that one step closer the next time around. In essence, we are the anchor.

Functions and *Meaning* of Behavior

Many schools have hired Board-Certified Behavior Analysts (BCBAs) to help "analyze" behavior, primarily looking at children through a strict behavioral lens. As a result, some positive changes have occurred, including more attention paid to student behavior overall, especially that which precedes challenging behavior (antecedents) as well as what reinforces that behavior (consequences). There is also greater emphasis on using data to measure whether their interventions are successful. These have been helpful steps. Some families, especially those who have children with autism or other developmental issues, also work with BCBAs at home.

Given this direction, there is a great deal of discussion about trying to understand the *functions* of behavior. Typically, these emphasize behaviors that are (1) attention seeking, (2) task avoidant/escape oriented, or (3) reflective of sensory/emotional dysregulation. Also noted are interpersonal skills deficits and behaviors due to medical concerns. For example, a child with Tourette's syndrome might interrupt by calling out a vocal or verbal tic, but this is neurologically driven rather than intentional behavior. It is, in the formal legal language of schools, behavior directly related to one's disability.

My concern, however, after reading many hundreds of reports, is that we sometimes funnel behaviors into these categories without understanding their *meaning*. Knowing that a child's actions are attention-seeking tells us only that, in effect, the child seeks attention. The question, of course, is *why* the child wants or needs attention. The story is incomplete without a working theory about what underlies that goal. Here's an example: A smart, remarkably insightful, and severely traumatized 8th-grade boy, Lawrence, once told me that, if he did not get an adult's "eyes on" him at least every 20 minutes or so, he'd begin, in his words, to "fall apart" with anxiety. For years, his loud, disruptive behavior had been classified—correctly, it turns out—as attention-seeking, but it had an entirely different reason underlying it. Rather than ignoring his attention-gathering behavior or removing him from class, another intervention made better sense: Teachers checked in with him approximately every 15 minutes, even if it meant just walking by his desk and tapping him on the shoulder. (He was not averse to touch.) Not one of his teachers reported this to be a burden and, with a different rationale about why he needed their attention, there was willingness, even an eagerness, to help. It was literally just this one single intervention that, for the most part, turned around his classroom behavior. (It also helped that his relationships took on a more positive tone.) I know we all wish that it was consistently this simple, which it certainly is not, but it points to how grasping the meaning behind the behavior, rather than just its function, can make a significant difference in both our understanding and how we intervene.

I have observed countless interventions that were based on adults counseled to ignore children's attention-seeing behavior. From a strictly behavioral perspective, this appears to make sense; avoid reinforcing negative behavior and then reward the positive (the non-attention-seeking) behavior. Sometimes, though, this is less than practical. If children will de-escalate on their own, this is a viable option; when another child will continue to escalate until things reach a crisis point and disrupt an entire classroom—the story of Lawrence is an example—planned ignoring is not at all useful. In short, to understand the meaning and subtleties of attention-seeking behavior is to develop more effective intervention strategies.

Task avoidance. Similarly, we need to know more when a child is labeled "task avoidant." What hypothesis do we hold as to the underlying reason? There are children who avoid tasks on purpose. Anxious, perfectionistic students may not start a task if they are concerned about making a mistake. Those with learning disabilities might choose to "mask" their learning struggles by either acting out or disappearing. (I know many such children who make regular visits to the bathroom or the nurse's office during specific academic classes.) A significant percentage of students with attention-deficit/hyperactivity disorder (ADHD) have a corresponding written-output disorder, and some will find any way possible to avoid performing any tasks related to writing. Depressed children may not have the energy, focus, or motivation to take on a challenging academic activity and will find ways around having to do it. This list goes on.

Sometimes our children, regardless of their psychological makeup and no matter the reason, simply do not want to do a particular activity. As noted economist John Kenneth Galbraith was quoted as saying, "One of the best ways of avoiding necessary and even urgent tasks is to seem to be busily employed on things that are already done." Lots of adults can utilize this skill when needed, but many children, especially those with less developed social awareness skills, do not know how. As such, they are forced to resort to less subtle and savvy methods. (And they are thus more likely to be caught in their evasion.) Avoidance, then, is not always a reflection of trauma or mental illness. Sometimes it represents nothing more than a child's reaction to a perceived lack of personal choice, but we commonly see it as a coping strategy in children who have PTSD.

Children with trauma may try to dodge tasks for all the reasons I just named. And for some, as noted, the idea of making a mistake in class is intertwined with being severely criticized or hurt for even the smallest errors made elsewhere, so they find ways to sidestep situations in which they perceive that any risk exists. There are few scenarios in which there is zero chance of making a mistake, especially in a learning environment, which helps to explain why some children with trauma find school painfully hard. Fortunately, there are also students with trauma who excel in school and have been able to compartmentalize their stress such that they will take some degree of risk in this setting. That is, they have been able, with or without help, to distinguish when it is safe to put themselves out there and launch into new challenges.

There are also traumatized children who *unintentionally* avoid tasks. This is an important distinction. Children stressed to the point of dissociation may shut down to the degree that they cannot mobilize themselves to focus or learn. Jessica, a 13-year-old with a history of physical and sexual abuse, reports that she shuts down so completely in some of her classes—especially those taught by men—that she needs to walk straight out of the classroom or she will become immobilized. This has been perceived by teachers and others in school as purposeful, defiant behavior, but her perspective is different: She views it as her only way to cope. Jessica envisions no other viable option in the moment. What this example reveals is that children with trauma will, by necessity, prioritize their internal sense of survival—the perception of safety—rather than rules or the demands of their teachers and principals or, at times, of their parents or guardians. It is only by recognizing the fundamental, evolutionary reality of fight, flight, or freeze and crafting a plan sensitive to a child's experience and needs that we will help the child make progress.

Continuing the discussion of avoidance, Fischer (2015) describes a well-known phenomenon referred to as Failure to Launch (FTL) syndrome. Not a formal diagnosis, it is more a depiction of what happens to avoidant children when they reach important transitional moments in their lives. This can mean anything from leaving home for kindergarten to departing for college, the military, or a job. Children with trauma often display FTL because their experience has taught them that it is not safe to change, try something new, take a risk, or deviate in any way from what they already know and understand. To me, their tendency to avoid is one of the more debilitating aspects of trauma. It means that they may have little sense that the future will be better than the present or the past. It is exactly here that we need to focus many of our efforts to help.

Sensory and emotional regulation. When you hear the phrase "sensory issues," what do you think of? Most people instantly identify autism. It is widely accepted that children with autism spectrum disorders have sensory overstimulation. This may be based on noise, touch, lights or other visual stimuli, or motion in a child's visual field (which defines recess, hall passing, and most typical educational settings, even in a normally active classroom). While the amount and impact may be debated, I have heard little dispute over this idea. Children with ADHD often present with similar challenges. Less frequently recognized is that children with trauma usually have comparable difficulties with managing sensory stimulation. We understand, for example, that soldiers returning from a war zone may jump at the sound of a backfiring car engine or a plane passing loudly overhead. This is not dysregulation caused by an organic condition; clearly, it is based on one's lived experience in an unpredictable, potentially dangerous environment. (In the military, returning soldiers who react this way were often diagnosed with "shell shock.") It is no different for children with trauma. I have witnessed children who will scream that another person's normal talking "hurts their ears" or that someone looking at them is like having a hole drilled through their skin; eye contact is sometimes portrayed in terms that can only be described as assaultive. I have seen others who will literally leap out of their seats if you approach them unexpectedly.

Here's another example: You had a difficult, stressful day at work; you were running behind the entire time; your dog got sick all over the house this morning; and one of your kids was in an irritable mood when you picked the child up late in the afternoon. You get home only to realize that you forgot to pick up what you needed to cook dinner. If you are like many of us, the sound of your kids' arguing is louder and more grating on days like this; the other drivers on the road seem more aggressive than ever; the lights seem brighter and more glaring; your patience is at best thin, and you want to shut out all ringing cell phones, beeping computers, and any other distractions.

This is what ordinary overstimulation feels like, although it does not feel so ordinary when you are in the middle of it. For children with trauma, some of whom have regularly coped by straining to stay vigilant and never letting their guard down (meaning they rarely, if ever, get to decompress), this is what life is like on a daily if not moment-to-moment basis. Thus, it should come as no surprise that many of these children are high-wired, on edge, exhausted, and living with chronic sensory overload. Their startle reflex may be dramatically high, which means that managing outside stimulation is an ongoing challenge. This in combination with their emotional strife and intrusive thoughts illuminates how challenging and stressful it is for children to live with trauma.

When you hear the words "emotional regulation," which diagnosis immediately comes to mind? Many of us—in fact, virtually everyone to whom I posed the question—name bipolar disorder right away. It is a logical choice since difficulty regulating one's emotions is a hallmark. The addition to the *DSM-5* of disruptive mood dysregulation disorder (DMDD) represents another diagnosis that signifies a child's ongoing irritability and anger. The struggle is similar for traumatized children, but it reflects their lived experience rather than solely a contribution from organic causes. In the nature-nurture balance, it is more about the latter (unless, of course, the child has other physiological, psychological, or developmental issues.) Because children with PTSD, especially when it derives from some form of abuse at home, have not been exposed to healthy coping skills, they are likely to lack good self-calming strategies. If we add in some degree of *hypervigilance*— relentlessly scanning their surroundings to make sure there is no imminent danger, even in situations where there is no trace of any—they are at risk of developing chronically high levels of irritability and moodiness. That means it is more challenging for them to maintain an even keel amid what they perceive as stressful situations. At times, it does not take much to set them off. We may complain that these children lack resilience, but it is apparent why this might be true.

Impact on learning: Traumatized children do not necessarily learn effectively—or comfortably—in how we traditionally teach in schools. Since both *maintaining* and *shifting* attention can be challenging, they may view a steady stream of different academic tasks as nearly impossible to accomplish. Also, as noted, many children with PTSD are hypervigilant, and therefore, they tend to pay attention to the wrong classroom cues; these children are attending to their fears, worries, and perceived threats rather than the academic content in front of them. Neuroscientists refer to the term *salience*, the ability to discern what is most important and relevant in any task. As I recently observed in both high school and 2nd-grade classrooms, a child can miss key points of what should be taken away from a specific learning activity. Traumatized children are often focused elsewhere; they may be mentally processing their experience rather than tuning into what is taking place in the moment. One child told me that all she thinks about is what happened before and what might happen in the future. This observation speaks clearly to the frustration many others express about trying to succeed in an academic setting. She is, in essence, absent from the here-and-now, which distracts her from any sustained learning and maintains, if not increases, her stress.

Another impact of trauma on learning is in the realm of *processing speed*. This, in short, is how efficiently one perceives auditory or visual information. The processing speed index, as it is known, is one of the five elements that, when measured, combine to indicate a child's IQ score. Neurodevelopment—our biology—is at the heart of whether someone has a sufficient processing speed, but emotional factors play a significant role as well. Anxiety slows processing speed. And since trauma is marked by anxiety, it makes sense that a child's processing speed would be slowed. Those of us who have ever been struck by a bout of anxiety, or multiple bouts, know firsthand that it can be hard to focus, to take in and make sense of new information, especially if it is coming at us quickly. This happens when we are fatigued as well.

If this sounds too vague, consider this: If you know a little bit of a second or, if you are fortunate, a third language, maybe you have had the experience of proudly utilizing your limited vocabulary with a native speaker. What may come back is a torrent of that same language with words, phrases, and idioms that make absolutely no sense to you. That deer-in-the-headlights look on your face (which would most certainly be mine) is a natural response to being overwhelmed by language. This is what the typical classroom experience is like for children with slow processing speed, especially if, in my experience, they score below the 10th percentile. One adolescent boy reported that the impact on his confidence and general sense of well-being in school was enormous, leaving him feeling humiliated and "stupid." I have consistently heard that latter word when children are revealing enough to share their self-perceptions. The inability to comprehend the nuances of language, to keep up with what is being said, is, in the words of another student, horrible and embarrassing.

The better news is that there are strategies for helping them. For one thing, many children benefit from knowing about their processing speed in a straightforward way. As such, it helps if the evaluator reviews their testing results directly with them. They need to know that their scores usually show that they are anything but "stupid" and that they just struggle in this specific area. I have witnessed vast relief from people of all ages who finally come to understand their struggle, especially when it is rooted in a discussion of their strengths. For children whose scores show that their learning challenges are more widespread, the story is similar: They deserve to know where their strengths lie and to have some context for understanding both their academic difficulties and any challenges in grasping the nuances of their various social interactions.

There is another way to help: In one study (Rowe, 1986), it was discovered that the average teacher waits nine-tenths seconds—that is, less than a single second—before moving on to another student or providing the answer. Given the fast pace of classroom instruction and the pressures teachers face due to standardized testing and other demands, it is hard to imagine that the amount of wait time has increased since Rowe published her findings. The recommendation is for a full three seconds. It may not sound like a lot of time, but classroom teachers live daily with the challenge of maintaining a consistent pace and the need to keep things moving so that they do not lose the attention of their other students during oral instruction or group discussions. For many students, however, and not just those with the slowest processing speed, it is necessary to have these added moments to make sense of what is being asked and then to formulate a response. (In the autism field, this is referred to as a lag in *throughput*, a term that makes a great deal of implicit sense. It is the concept that some children can take in information but need extra time to make sense of it and translate their thoughts into action.) With those students who are unable to successfully process directions within the larger group, it helps to strategize about ways the teacher can make sure they understand instructions without losing face in front of their peers. Most teachers I interact with are committed to making sure these students do not fear that they are drowning in their classrooms; at the same time, teachers are actively searching for tools to help with the process.

Living with trauma is often marked by depression, just as it is by anxiety. A hallmark of depression is difficulty with what is known as *initiation*, the formal term for saying simply that someone is having trouble getting started with an activity. (We often see a similar picture in children with traumatic brain injuries, or TBIs.) It is clear how this would affect children's performance in the classroom: If children struggle to get started, the anxiety and panic build up, and suddenly they are angry or shutting down rather than attending to the activity, even one that they can normally handle. Although at times it has taken some convincing, there are teachers willing to help such students begin tasks, whether it is to write the first two words of a sentence or sketch out the first steps in a math problem. Doing so is almost like getting a boulder moving down the hill: The momentum picks up and accelerates. But teachers have to overcome the understandable worry that they are hindering a child's independence. In this scenario, independence is a relative concept, and if that child can complete a task after just a bit of help at the outset, it is a useful trade-off. Some children, once they develop more confidence in any specific classroom, have a lessening need for this help. Without it, though, a lot of power struggles and hurt feelings ensue, often for both student and teacher.

As noted, avoidance is another hallmark of trauma. Trying to stay away from any possibility of making a mistake leaves children with the magical but false belief that they cannot be hurt or that they will be protected from feeling any of the range of painful emotions. But, just as with anxiety, the more one avoids, the more one's energy goes toward remaining unengaged, whether this refers to school, friends, family, or participation in any sort of activity. In short, it is a kind of shutting down of experience, an understandable attempt at coping but one with consequences that reduce a child's basic quality of life. In the realm of learning, it means that a child may resolutely take no risks or refuse to go beyond anything but the most concrete yes or no answers. On our end, educators can be instrumental in helping these students by finding ways to maintain a meaningful connection in the face of this sometimes very direct stay away message. Once children learn that "the world won't end," as one child put it, when they make the inevitable academic mistake, they can begin to move toward more active learning. Admittedly, depending on the child, it can be a lengthy and time-consuming process to reach this point.

Finally, low frustration tolerance and a lack of resilience can be major barriers to learning. As noted, children with trauma frequently struggle over making errors and bouncing back. Despite our encouraging words, they may not know how to move on after hitting a roadblock. One adolescent told me that her thoughts begin "churning" when she perceives that she is struggling over an academic activity or worrying that an impending one will be too hard. So she fails, she says, "fully, totally and completely." She also uses the phrase "drop right to the bottom" to describe her inability to turn things around once she senses a possible failure. This is common among children with trauma histories, but it can lead to serious complications. Without a working idea of how to rebound, many children go into fight, flight, or freeze in these moments. A primary goal of teaching social-emotional learning (SEL) is to help children develop greater "grit" and perseverance, even in light of making a mistake or a poor choice. For many children with trauma, learning how to overcome challenges—to develop resilience and self-regulation—is the skill area they need to develop most of all.

In the realm of SEL, currently a common phrase and area of concern among school districts across the United States, there are five core areas to consider: self-awareness, self-management, social awareness (which relates to the capacity for empathy), relationship skills, and responsible decision-making (Collaborative for Academic, Social and Emotional Learning, or CASEL, 2019). Given the discussion in this chapter, it should be clear how each of these might be affected by a child's history of trauma. These are of course developmental challenges for all children, which underlies why many schools have begun to integrate SEL thinking into their overall curriculum. The challenges are only magnified for traumatized children. Later chapters will further amplify this statement and explore how the different aspects of SEL need to be addressed.

Each of the elements discussed in this chapter—lack of trust, avoidance, the need for predictability, relationship problems, learning differences, and challenging behaviors—lends itself to recognizing that academic demands and, notably, the relational aspects of school are inherently stressful for many children with trauma. Given the amount of time and energy devoted to trying to help them "manage" their behaviors and, ultimately, to support their growth, we need to develop a solid framework for how to sustain these children. Going forward, our sweeping awareness that all areas of children's lives are affected—their social interactions, behaviors, emotions, and learning and attentional skills—is crucial to building in the right kinds of help. There can be no healing presence without this.

CHAPTER TWO

Support Planning and the Basic Pyramid

Before I launch into a discussion of my Pyramid model, here are some relevant data to indicate why such a model is needed. Numbers provided by the National Survey of Children's Health for 2016 were unexpectedly high, revealing that almost half of the children in the United States have suffered at least one traumatic event, which translates to an astonishing 34,000,000 children. The same survey found that almost one-third of children between the ages of 12 and 17 have experienced two or more kinds of serious childhood adversity, meaning more than 8,000,000 children. Of children and adolescents overall, 3% to 15% of girls and 1% to 6% of boys develop PTSD (National Center for PTSD). The National Institute of Mental Health found more specific numbers falling within that same range: 7% of girls and 2% of boys diagnosed with PTSD.

There is not another diagnosis in the entire *Diagnostic and Statistical Manual (DSM-5)* that suggests the possibility of such a wide range. In other words, the term gets deployed, if not loosely, then at least with a lack of diagnostic clarity. We need to more clearly understand what we mean by *trauma* before applying the term directly to any specific child. While we may not know exactly how many children are suffering, we do know with certainty that it is not a small number. Personally, and similar to other experienced clinicians I know, I use an approximate figure of somewhere between 3% and 4% of all children. No matter the actual percentage, it is large enough that some researchers are urging the United States to view trauma as a public health crisis (Copeland et al., 2018).

If we needed further evidence of trauma's terrible impact, the link between childhood trauma and suicide is well established in the existing research. DeRubeis et al. (2016) found that there is a "potent" connection between trauma and both suicidal ideation and actual attempts. More specifically, child sexual abuse directly contributes to suicidal behavior (O'Brien & Sher, 2013). The National Survey of Children's Behavior (U.S. Census Bureau, 2017) found that children diagnosed with PTSD are *15 times* more likely to attempt suicide. These findings contradict observations that these children are simply out to get their own way; I frequently hear them described as "selfish," "self-absorbed," and "manipulative" when "suffering" and "self-hating" might be the more apt terms. As we will discuss, trauma is not an excuse for disruptive behavior, but it certainly helps explain it in many cases. With suicide rates increasing dramatically in the United States, especially among boys and young men of color (see the website of Centers for Disease Control and Prevention: https://www.cdc.gov/injury/wisqars/index.html; Curtin & Heron, 2019), Copeland et al.'s description of trauma as a public health crisis should be seen as a literal call to action.

A thought-provoking distinction between *suffering* and *adversity* was articulated by one of the participants, a woman, in the documentary *Any One of Us* (2019), which tells the story of people recovering from spinal cord injuries. The woman, who spent many years in a wheelchair, describes *suffering* as "having to endure." She contrasts this with *adversity*, either something or a series of events that one has the potential to overcome through hard work, belief, and unyielding effort. Grief underlies both. In adversity, these are not mutually exclusive states of being: One can continue to grieve a loss of any kind, whether it is the capacity to move physically or the safe relationship one desperately wished for, and still hold fast to the belief that life can get better.

PTSD seems to coincide with notions of *both* suffering and adversity. The balance depends on the child—the child's temperament, support system, and philosophical and religious beliefs as well as the child's history—as there is often deep suffering carried with the adversity that results from traumatizing life events. I am struck that the goal for all of us is to help children, at their own pace, shift from a state of suffering—enduring—toward viewing their world in terms of facing the adverse situations they have encountered. In the latter, there is more hope and more possibility for action. This is where the Pyramid model comes in. While it does not ignore a child's suffering, it reflects that terrible events happen and yet there is still a way forward.

The *Basic Pyramid*. In responding to a crisis, the most effective way to combat chaos is to focus on bringing order and structure to whatever the situation might be. That is, stabilization is the first order of business in a true emergency, whether it is an individual having a mental health emergency, a home in disarray, or a large city torn apart by a hurricane. This kind of thinking underlies the Basic Pyramid, a model that can be applied in a wide range of situations. (I will generally refer to the model as "the Pyramid.")

Because traumatized children can at times act in ways that disrupt themselves as well as their peers, teachers, and caregivers, my goal was to develop a tool that could contribute to creating and maintaining a calmer, less reactive environment. For adults, stress is often determined by not knowing what to do in a situation; the Pyramid is an attempt to clarify the steps to be taken both before and during the time a child escalates so that everyone can approach the situation with more confidence and less stress. Typically, the calmer the adults around them, the quicker children will begin to de-escalate.

Whether we are reacting to a child's behavioral and emotional crisis or doing our best to prevent one, we are, according to one middle school principal, "desperate to find measures that work." To address traumatized children's needs, then, why a pyramid and not, for example, a triangle? Or some other shape? And why does it even matter? A pyramid suggests something solid. It has a sturdy base. It narrows as it moves skyward, just as this intervention model does, but it retains a needed sense of permanence. According to Bhengu (2014), "The ancient Egyptians saw the shape of the pyramids as a method of providing new life . . . because the pyramid represented the form of the physical body emerging from the earth and ascending towards the light of the sun." He goes on to say that, on the spiritual level, the pyramid is both a symbol of "integration" and "harmony," which are components usually lacking in children who have been traumatized. This, then, seems the perfect structure to represent our efforts to help.

I conceive of the Pyramid as a *redesign* and organizing structure rather than an entirely novel creation. It may be that the difference is narrow or no more than intellectual hairsplitting. Whatever the case, many ideas for how to help struggling children have been floated, but I have not encountered a well-defined, comprehensive approach that can be used in schools, homes, and other settings. The approach adopted here is based on understanding trauma, carefully identifying the developmental needs and abilities of each child, recognizing the significance of a child's environment, and then shaping our interventions differently than we have historically done. And it acknowledges the critical yet time-consuming need for collaboration, follow-up, and thorough consideration of the impact of our interventions. Along with all these elements, we have to be organized and structured in how we develop the Pyramid. To integrate this kind of thinking into ongoing school processes will ensure at least a greater likelihood for success. It is a serious commitment but one well worth making.

All the considerations in the first chapter having to do with the intricacies of *relationship*—trust, predictability, how the child connects with adults—must be factored into any plan of action. Otherwise, we run the risk of being driven by the model rather than steered by the needs of a specific child. While the Pyramid provides a comprehensive, uncomplicated approach, it must be used flexibly and with common sense. If it doesn't pass the so-called eyeball test in any specific situation, then it has been implemented poorly and should be reviewed. Applying the model is where careful planning, creativity, and collaboration are required. At the same time, we need to develop a working hypothesis about the child's behavior and emotional world to braid together the entire process.

This model, which I refer to broadly as a "support plan," is based on three steps (see figure 2.1). It was unintentional, but the steps roughly fall in line with the Response to Intervention (RTI) model, part of the Multi-Tiered Systems of Support (MTSS) approach now commonly used in school districts. That is, each step (or "tier" in RTI language) progresses logically to the next, more intensive stage if the prior intervention (or set of interventions) has been unsuccessful.

The first step is *prevention*. This is the thickest area of the Pyramid and the part upon which the rest of the plan rests. An overarching aspect of prevention is this: It is essential to consider what triggers a child to enter the negative spiral of acting out or shutting down. This can be challenging to determine, and it takes time and patience to develop hypotheses. Some children can help us with this exploration; others cannot or will not. No matter what the triggers are, and whether they are a constant in upsetting the child, it is important to remember that children with trauma tend to mislabel the level of risk in various situations. At times, they may perceive threat where none exists. This is a common factor, one that happens almost across the board for children who have been abused. Any efforts at prevention have to account for it.

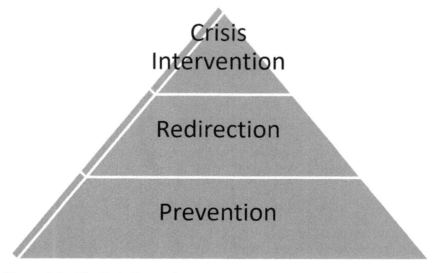

Figure 2.1   The Basic Pyramid

Van der Kolk (2014) refers to this as an "alarm system" gone awry. Similarly, Kahneman (2011) describes what he calls "System 1 thinking," a way of processing information neurologically that is rapid and emotionally based such that there is an almost automatic response to how one perceives an event. The extension of his concept is that, based on a painful emotional encounter (or a series of them), any child is likely to become inflamed by events, people, or memories associated in some way with that experience. We should not be surprised, then, by a traumatized child's apparent misperception of or overreaction to a negative interaction or incident. And it is exactly the reason why we need a support plan in place.

For any child with trauma—although I certainly use the model with nontraumatized children with serious emotional and behavioral struggles as well—I ask teachers (as well as parents and other caregivers) to identify three to five preventive strategies that *might work* for the child *some of the time*. Since everyone needs to participate in the problem-solving process knowing that no single intervention or specific set of strategies will always be successful, it is important to emphasize that we are trying to craft as broad a repertoire of preventive approaches as possible, not aiming for a magical fix. Even by asking the question, we can begin to shift the focus to thinking about what skills the child needs to develop rather than emphasizing what the child has done wrong.

If teachers cannot identify more than a single preventive strategy that might work for a child who is struggling, I ask school counselors to try to explore additional options. It does not have to be a lengthy process, just a thoughtful one that carefully accounts for the nature of that child. Typically, this can be done in two to four short meetings. As an example, for aggressive or explosive students, I prefer to schedule in their breaks from the classroom rather than wait until they either earn them or are too late in receiving them. In the language of behaviorists, these breaks are "noncontingent." This keeps children's stress from spiraling to a level where they are more likely to break down.

There is ongoing debate about the value of sensory integration approaches to help children self-regulate. I do not plan to enter into that discussion, because the literature is mixed and not definitive. What I do know is that some simple sensory interventions can be successful for the right child in the right situation. For example, I observed a 10-year-old boy who consistently slid over from his assigned spot on the rug to burrow his two feet into the soft chair in which his teacher sat during a group read-aloud activity. Despite repeated requests to stop, the behavior continued, generally after a break of 15 or 20 seconds. It was off-putting to the teacher, but though she clearly viewed it as noncompliance—this was not new behavior—she was open to trying an experiment. We seated this child in a chair with a bungee cord strung across the bottom legs. (Occupational therapists have frequently used such an approach, so there was nothing particularly novel about it other than, perhaps, that in this case it was for a child identified with PTSD rather than ADHD, autism, or sensory integration disorder.) The difference was immediate: This boy listened to the story while happily kicking his feet against the cord; and when he was asked a question, he was able to provide a response, showing that he was paying attention. None of the other students was interrupted by his behavior. Thus emerged an ideal form of prevention that was simple, not disruptive or time-consuming, and it did not include either removal from the classroom or the need for a reward system. Again, if it was only this easy more of the time.

Mindfulness has become a popular tool in schools (Maynard, Solis, Miller, & Brendel, 2017). Many children benefit from a reminder to breathe and to quietly note both their surroundings and their internal sensations in the present moment. However, some children with trauma will become increasingly agitated—more anxious, more heightened—if they focus on their breathing or their internal state, especially if they have not had enough practice and feedback first. If they are inhaling rapidly or beginning to hyperventilate, they may be unable to apply strategies for slowing down, which adds to their distress. Not long ago, I witnessed a child, probably 12 years old, who went into a full-blown panic attack when encouraged to "focus on your breathing." I also had a conversation with a child who has asthma along with his PTSD who had been encouraged to count his breaths in and out up to six, which made him anxious and precipitated an asthma attack. Clearly, this strategy does not work for everyone. The *what works* needs to be explored with the child during calmer times, outside of crisis moments. That is when a child's problem-solving capacities are at their most accessible. Usually, this process of exploration is led by a school counselor; teachers can then follow up with reminders for the child to apply those newly-developing coping skills.

Some children benefit from progressive muscle relaxation strategies that can be easily adapted for the classroom. For example, I ask traumatized children to squeeze and release one or two fingers on their opposite hand (repeating eight to 10 times); anecdotally, I would say that about half find it calming—they note that the muscles in their arms and then their shoulders and neck begin to soften—and the other half report it has no effect at all. A number of children are drawn to using old-fashioned isometric exercises such as repeatedly squeezing their palms together and then releasing. Others are more comfortable with something known as "chair push-ups," in which they simply do a push-up-type motion using the arms of a chair. This illustrates why children need the opportunity to try out different options in a safe setting before attempting to apply them during high-stress moments. I find that many children, including adolescents when they are willing to "go there," are motivated to find tools that work for them. Occupational therapists are often uniquely skilled in helping to develop a menu of these sensorimotor interventions, but counselors can do the same.

It is similar with visualization strategies. Conjuring an image of a peaceful scene or a safe person works for a fair number of children; some will calm their bodies and refocus. You can almost watch their shoulders loosen as they begin to wind down. Others, however, will be thrown off by attempting to visualize. Children have explained to me that they could not access their comforting visualizations when under stress or that they could not even remember what those visualizations were. Some children become frightened and upset just by closing their eyes around other people. The difficulties—often described, in these children's minds, in the language of failure—only made them feel worse and more destabilized. If we need another reminder, it is that these tools are child-specific and require practice if they are to be helpful.

I find that physical movement, more than almost any other single form of prevention, is markedly helpful in comforting a child. There is a good reason why child therapists pound out so many miles of walking with their clients; movement soothes the nervous system, and since both adult and child are looking in front of them, it removes the intensity of eye contact and allows the child a better sense of control and safety. I find that children seem more fluid in their thinking and speaking; many of them report just that, including one boy who told me he becomes "clearer in his head" afterward. It has been long established that exercise is a useful antidote to anxiety and depression and is healthy for the brain (Ratey & Manning, 2014). Finding ways to build this into the school day, beyond recess and physical education, is something that schools can do; I watched a teacher create, reluctantly at first, space and time for intermittent movement breaks within her classroom, which, she happily reported, decreased a significant buildup of tension among many of her students. The students included two boys with severe trauma histories, one of whom stretched vigorously and with such incredible and natural ease that I suspect he could be a future yoga master if he so chose.

For some children, brisk walking or even running laps helps. I worked with one child in a clinic setting who, when upset, would take me for laps around the rectangular clinic hallway. This boy could move fast. Run-walking was the most effective way for him to calm his nervous system, and after a while, we decided together to start our sessions this way. We did not knock over anyone else brave enough to prowl the hallways—that is how I remember it, anyway—and I recall that as he gradually slowed his pace, he would tell me he was "ready for the office." At other times, while seated in a chair or on the floor, he would suddenly launch himself into doing jumping jacks, for him a reliable way to manage stress and maintain his focus on difficult topics. We had many in-depth conversations while he leapt up and down and I attempted to keep my disorientation at bay.

Another approach to prevention entails using a traditional five- or 10-point scale. Some school counselors have adapted these from the pain scales used in doctors' offices and emergency rooms and ask children to "grade" their level of anxiety. I use them with children to address their stress, level of anger, or even their ability to attend. (Those with ADHD often do well with the latter, but children with trauma, who may be distracted by their internal thoughts, also can benefit.) Some students take to this right away, others struggle with it, and there are those who are unable or unwilling to engage in such a reflective, inward-looking task. When it works for a specific child, however, it can be invaluable. I saw a 15-year-old girl gradually shift from being overwhelmed nearly all the time to someone who could slow down enough to assess her level of stress and then apply various strategies that she had rehearsed, especially a specific breathing technique that she took to almost right away. (Inhale to the count of four, exhale to the count of four; inhale to four, exhale to six; inhale to four, exhale to eight; then repeat the sequence.) Until that time, she had never stopped to consider how much stress she was under and how it might affect her in the moment. It brought about a significant improvement in her well-being. In addition, many schools now use the Zones of Regulation program (Kuypers, 2011), which aims to help children develop greater awareness of their internal mood states and, as a result, increase their level of self-control.

A different approach to prevention is based on how adults think about and interact with children. Adopting a developmental mindset rather than a fixed-trait one can make a significant difference. Early-childhood educators tend to think in the former and, as a result, they often use language such as "the child is so far unable to . . ." or "it's hard for the child right now" rather than "the child won't" or "the child refuses to." Perhaps this sounds like a subtle distinction and a minor intervention, but such a perspective—and thus the wording we use when talking directly with children—can help alleviate the stress and sense of being not good enough that traumatized children often carry. Many children with trauma are acutely attuned to messages of failure; our own change in mindset can contribute to changing theirs.

Any trauma-informed approach, no matter which one, must emphasize prevention and, as part of this, must teach self-regulation (and, by extension, coping) skills. The Pyramid embraces this idea, and in practice, it is essential that schools, and any other setting in which there are ongoing interactions with children with trauma, incorporate a regular planning-and-review process to develop and implement the most effective prevention methods for any specific child. There is much discussion about being "proactive" in schools and other organizations; this process alone is a giant stride in that direction. It is the same on the home front, no matter whom the child lives with.

The second step in the Pyramid is *redirection*. The goal here is to help children shift their attention from whatever is triggering their upset to a different focus. Asking an open-ended question such as "What's wrong?" is typically not successful in these moments, especially for children who struggle to identify their internal states. Sometimes, with younger children, it can be as simple as making a request to "please get something for me." For other children, a quick movement break—especially if done together with an adult—offers a release from their negative thoughts and emotions. This is where the early stages of de-escalation come in, especially if a child tends to become aggressive. A quiet voice, a warm tone, a reassuring look: I have seen each of these work across many tense situations.

In therapy-speak we refer to this process as *co-regulation*. Children who cannot or are struggling to self-regulate—meaning, essentially, that they cannot calm their nervous systems to the point where they can think and problem-solve clearly—benefit from the presence of an adult who can provide that source of comfort and anchoring. It is an amazing sight to behold when an agitated child begins to relax and "come down" in the face of someone who can model and sustain a sense of calm. For some children, touch works to settle them; for others, though, especially those with histories of sexual and physical abuse, touch can make things worse, so it is critical to know with whom this can be used safely.

This idea of co-regulation also speaks to why time-outs typically do not work with traumatized children. A time-out may reduce the overstimulation inherent in being around a group of other children, but it also forces a child to be alone who may not have the self-calming skills to handle this. As a result, I frequently see children who become increasingly agitated when "put in time-out." The resulting lack of control, and the fact of no one there to help redirect a child's thoughts and emotions, often leads to further agitation. The presence of an adult, even one who is not initially speaking or interacting directly with the child, tends to work more effectively. Overall, this approach speaks to a view of trauma as something to work with—self-management skills needing to be developed—rather than a set of behaviors requiring discipline. Later, we will discuss restitution, the idea of making up for one's behaviors when they negatively affect others.

I ask children if they are able to offer suggestions as to what might help them shift from their negative thoughts to more of a problem-solving orientation. (I go to great lengths not to sound as though I am blaming them, emphasizing that I only want to help them find a less painful way to cope.) They respond in various ways to this request for solution-focused thinking: Some have useful recommendations, others have none, and a sizable number of them do not necessarily comprehend my question and look at me with confusion. This opens to a conversation about what redirection is and why it is a useful tool. At that point, I typically speculate aloud various possibilities and share what appears to work at times for other students. Clearly, there is no established protocol for how to do this, but I have often been surprised by the insights that children can provide.

The need for redirection is based on the reality that many children with trauma get locked into what is upsetting them and cannot alter their cata-strophic thinking. One woman with a lengthy trauma history told me that, during childhood, her painful self-judgments overwhelmed her ability to think rationally. She also struggled with intrusive negative thoughts that would appear without warning or specific reason. If children cannot transi-tion away from those thoughts on their own, then an external reminder—to move their physical selves, to draw a picture or use clay, to use a breathing, visualization, or progressive muscle relaxation strategy—has the best chance to redirect them before they reach a crisis point. One girl asked me to tell the adults in her life that a simple, short comment such as "It's time" would cue her that she was getting too locked in and needed to try to rebalance herself.

Early on, we create a menu of as many potentially successful strategies as possible so teachers and caregivers feel comfortable with how to proceed and so children can quickly try to access these tools. The best ones are those that they can use right in the classroom rather than having to transition to another location. Just as how children learn math and other academic skills via scaffolded steps, so should we expect a gradual shift rather than a dra-matic change in how successfully they self-regulate.

A common thread among children with severe trauma histories is that, when they become oppositional or shut down, they often find it difficult to "turn it around." A valuable problem-solving dialogue is one in which these children begin to recognize the pattern and work on strategies to keep them from "plummeting" all the way to the bottom. School counselors, and outside therapists as well, can be instrumental in this process. The idea that a prob-lem can "stay small and not grow into a huge mountain," as one girl expressed it to me, is sometimes a radical realization. This does not come easily to a number of children. It takes practice, sometimes a great deal of it.

The ability to turn it around is *resilience* in action. It also reflects *grit*, another word we hear regularly. These two terms are now firmly rooted in the cultural discussion of what children are said to need to develop to be suc-cessful in life. For those with trauma, those qualities are imperative. One teacher, describing a student diagnosed with PTSD, has shared that it is like "watching the wheels come off" when this boy makes even a minor mistake and then begins spiraling out of control. Learning how to check himself, to keep his internal alarm system from fully going off, is a challenge he is just beginning to undertake. In an alternative classroom I worked with for almost 17 years, the language of "you can turn it around" was a daily aspect of our discussions with children; it was both a useful reminder to them and a sign of encouragement and hope. To be clear, we also talked a great deal about *how* a child could turn it around, which is specific to each one.

Redirection, then, is about helping children who are "stuck." I use this language specifically, because talking with a child about getting "unstuck," and sharing that there are tools to help with this, is nonjudgmental, optimistic, and generally consistent with their impressions of what is happening. Children often describe their experience in just this way, without necessarily having an exact word for it. Sometimes I hear the word "trapped." Knowing there is a language that speaks to their experience and that there are possible ways out of this kind of paralysis can bring great relief. And, strategically, it can avert an oncoming crisis when successful. This is exactly the purpose of redirection, to stem the crisis before it emerges.

For adults, redirecting a child is a skill to develop. It is not necessarily one fully in place when we begin teaching, working as school administrators or, for that matter, parenting. We often respond out of our own emotions and experiences. So we have to observe our internal reactions with curiosity and an open mind. This allows us to more fully understand the child and what works and what does not. If we are too quick to respond in anger or to withdraw, it leaves little opportunity to actively engage the child and help the child get back on track. Any of us can get set off by certain comments or behaviors. Self-awareness, which can only be achieved through a willingness to reflect honestly on our own tendencies and style of relating, goes a long way to helping us maintain the even level of intensity we need to redirect a child in those moments.

Redirection is a critical (and sometimes underused) step in the Pyramid. At times, I see a sudden lurch into crisis when preventive strategies were not immediately successful. Redirection, the second phase shown in the Pyramid, attempts to interrupt this spiral and slow down the entire process; when successful, it brings the child back to awareness and the ability to think through a problem. This, of course, is exactly the goal.

The third step in the Pyramid is *crisis intervention*. There is good reason for this section to be the narrowest. As noted, everyone, including the child, should have a grasp of the crisis plan if the initial stages of prevention and redirection are not successful. Taking too many steps has the potential to be confusing, and the goal is to provide as clear and uncluttered a path as possible. Effective crisis intervention depends on everyone knowing what to do in the moment without having to delve into a stressful, drawn-out problem-solving process. In other words, the middle of a crisis is not the time to have to figure it out.

MacDonald (2016) describes three types of crises. These are (1) developmental, (2) situational, and (3) existential. *Developmental crises* are those that arise from some of the expected transitions in life, such as leaving home for the first time to attend school. *Situational crises* are related to specific moments and scenarios that overwhelm a person's ability to problem-solve and cope. *Existential crises* entail questions of whether a child feels a sense of belonging, a sense of importance to someone else, and in some cases, whether the child feels worthwhile or even, as one boy wondered earnestly, if he should be "allowed to live."

It is not hard to see how each of these three different categories of crisis might be relevant to children with severe trauma. They may have a crisis that represents one, two, or all three of these areas. Whatever the underlying reason, children may present as angry, impulsive, intimidating (if not outwardly threatening), anxious, avoidant, shut down, or any combination of these moods and behaviors. One adolescent explained crisis in this way: "It's like you're being sucked underwater. You keep going deeper and the water keeps getting higher above you. You're drowning. It's terrifying."

There is no sense of being in control or able to make thoughtful decisions. This is an overarching theme reported by vast numbers of people who have experienced abuse. Every child has a unique course of PTSD and expresses that trauma through different combinations of emotion, behavior, physical expression, ability to learn, and social skill. In spite of all this variation, I find that the inability to trust others and the lack of perceived control are two of the most commonly reported outcomes during and after a period of crisis. There can also be enormous waves of anxiety if the individual has not become numb and gone into a dissociative state.

If we are going to look at the specifics of how to intervene during crisis situations, we should start with a brief discussion of "relationship building." We often talk about this subject in schools and other caregiver settings. Like the word *trauma*, we see the term everywhere. We know it is important, but how to attend to it, to develop it concretely, to determine if we are making progress—these are harder pieces of the puzzle. During a severe crisis, when a traumatized child's reasoning and perspective-taking skills usually shut down (some of the very SEL skills we try to teach), we may witness that child become aggressive, which is an evolutionary fear response, or run away. Again, this is the fight, flight, or freeze concept in action. Having a strong, trusting relationship with a child does not fully stop this from happening but can help it occur less often and, hopefully, with less of a five-alarm overreaction. When individual children have at least one close adult relationship in a school, that person's presence alone can shorten the amount of time it takes for those children to regain their bearings, self-control, and reasoning abilities. This comes about often but not always; it is important for the adult to try to avoid taking either outcome personally.

Relationship building is critical, and yet, for some children, it is not necessarily an organic response to the presence of a kind, well-meaning adult. Along with building our own skills in this realm, we need to constantly work at it, check in with the child, accept the get-close-and-pull-away phenomenon, and be clear with our limits, boundaries, and expectations. When these pieces are in place, we can help a frightened, angry, hurting child begin to shift to a steadier, more trusting position. As we know, relationships are fluid, so there needs to be continued reflection by teams and individuals as to what is working and what is not. This can be challenging, especially given schools' historical mission centered almost exclusively on academic and vocational progress. But when one accepts the idea that relationship building and academic progress go hand in hand, this becomes less of an either/or argument. In short, we need both.

The significance of relationship building with children cannot be overstated, although I have occasionally seen puzzled or even glazed looks when discussing this during workshops or school consultations. It is almost as if we—educators, clinicians, and caregivers—assume we know how to do this effectively. But there is little evidence to support this position; we generally rely on our own perception of "how it's going." Duncan, Miller, Wampold, and Hubble (2010), for example, reveal that therapists, often assumed to be the most relationally astute of professionals, are surprisingly unrealistic in making assumptions about the strength of their relationships with clients. The researchers discovered this by, simply, surveying therapy clients when they were not in the presence of their clinical providers.

If we are going to talk about the importance of relationship building, we need to take honest note of the many pressures teachers face. Anyone who does this work knows how challenging it is to attend to academic demands, new school initiatives, curriculum changes, and the increasing demand to help children with their personal lives. Relationship building with traumatized children requires much in the way of energy and time, both of which can be hard to find. This is similar to what I hear from overwhelmed caregivers at home, that the ideas make sense but follow-through is demanding and sometimes grueling. I do not want to ignore these challenges, and it is essential to account for them when asking people to maintain their focus on the relational aspects of working with children. Santoro (2018) points to the "demoralization" of many teachers and suggests it is this very issue that underlies why so many choose to leave the profession. These ideas reinforce why it is important to provide a structure for achieving stronger relationships and helping children at every phase, including during their moments of crisis.

A report from *Education Week* (Sparks, 2019), referring to an intriguing study conducted by researchers at the University of Southern California and Bank Street College, found that cutting-edge work is being done to understand what happens in the brains of "top teachers" as they engage with students. Increasing our knowledge base for how to interact with seriously hurting students, and replicating successful approaches, will only improve our capacity to help and teach these children. This is exactly the goal of the study, which uses fMRI (functional magnetic resonance imaging) machines, interviews, and various physiological sensors to learn more about what underlies teachers highly proficient in connecting with their students. It is not something in which we are automatically adept, nor is it necessarily taught as part of educators' formal training, but we now recognize it as a crucial skill intrinsic to becoming a successful educator or caregiver.

In addition, the need for our ongoing and deepening awareness of children's differences in race, ethnicity, socioeconomic status, religion, gender, and gender identity cannot be isolated from a meaningful discussion of relationship building. Disability status and physical appearance matter as well. We should not discount the role these factors play in causing high stress levels and at times, affecting children's capacity to trust authority figures in their schools and communities. We know, for example, that, for Black children, having even *one* same-race teacher during elementary school increases their "educational attainment" (Gershenson, Hart, Hyman, Lindsay, & Papageorge, 2018). The researchers found that, significantly, this means they are more likely to graduate from high school and enroll in college. Talking about difference on the macro, or global, level is essential, but this discussion has to extend to how we understand any specific child who is struggling right in front of us.

Viewed through an ecological or biopsychosocial lens, issues of inequality, oppression and, at times, subtle or even outright discrimination underlie many instances of trauma. More specifically, some students are traumatized by dealing with those in power, especially if those adults are of a different race (Comas-Díaz, 2016). The National Child Traumatic Stress Network (2017) refers to this directly as "racial trauma," which it differentiates from "historical" and other forms of trauma. Therefore, paying consistent attention to relationship building, whether a child looks like us or not (maybe *especially* if a child does not look like us), takes on added importance as a way not only to combat specific instances of trauma but, more broadly, to emphasize social justice.

What does all this mean for building a coherent crisis intervention plan? It says that the quality of a child's relationships matters even at the narrowest, most concrete portion of the pyramid. And it suggests that we need to maintain our focus on de-escalation. This can only occur if we emphasize trying to support the child; we do this by staying quiet and contained in ourselves rather than matching the intensity of the child's mood or threatening consequences, such as suspension or, for younger children, even just the loss of recess time. In this context, physical safety—for the student, but for everyone else as well—is the priority. I have seen threats lead to acts of serious posturing if not outright aggression. One nine-year-old smashed through a wall with her fists and, before I even laid eyes on her, she threw her boots so hard that they literally whistled past my head as I walked into her classroom. If the adult cannot model self-control and presence of mind, the child will escalate further. This is not necessarily easy to do in a stress-filled moment, but it is crucial. And it is what has the greatest likelihood of success. Any discussion of consequences or what will happen to the child as a result of the child's behavior needs to wait. This point cannot be overstated.

Support does not necessarily require a lot of talk. Fewer words are far more effective when someone is having difficulty making sense of next steps or thinking things through in a meaningful way. As noted, processing speed often slows when someone is under significant stress. I have noted with interest that many of us talk even more rapidly, and sometimes more loudly, when an agitated child begins to escalate or shut down. This, of course, only widens the gap between what we are trying to communicate and what the child can take in, leading to frustration and anxiety for both.

Similarly, it helps to offer a limited number of structured options to an agitated child—either "this" or "that"—rather than open-ended choices, which only taxes the child's problem-solving abilities and often leads to more escalation. It is not necessarily an intuitive approach, but it tends to generate less stress and outright opposition. I let the child who cannot make a choice know that I will wait, at least until I think the child is ready to take a step in one direction or another.

Juan, an 11-year-old boy whose mother vanished overnight and sent word that he should live with his grandmother instead, was devastated by her sudden abandonment of him. Nightmares, flashback memories of his mother, and disruptive behaviors appeared. He had until this time been a rather quiet, friendly boy. Predictably, things changed quickly, and school staff were concerned about how to both support him and set reasonable expectations for his behavior. Since he would quickly go into crisis, which meant loud yelling and occasional head banging, the crisis intervention plan, which Juan understood, was geared to teachers asking him to either "go over to the quiet area with me" or "walk with me to the counselor's office." This was done quietly, with no more words than these. After a few moments, Juan typically was able to choose one or the other, although it sometimes took more than one request before he could respond. The fact that he had already established good relationships with his teachers no doubt helped the process.

Counselors and principals are sometimes criticized for "coddling" children who act out in class. I have spoken with countless teachers who complain that these students get to "play games" outside the room without consequence and then simply return to class. (Sometimes, they report, these children are not necessarily ready to settle back into task demands.) Whether those nonclassroom staff articulate a trauma-informed philosophy or not, their approach is consistent with this kind of thinking. It prioritizes defusing a child over worrying about immediate consequences, which is a plus. The problem, however, is that we may miss certain sticking points about sending the child back to class: Is the child able to handle the stimulation of the class-room? Can the child successfully transition from preferred activities to class-room demands? Is the child able to organize thinking and problem-solving skills enough to consider what strategies to use to cope better upon return-ing? What is the history for this child in going back into the classroom after an emotional and/or behavioral crisis? To me, the philosophy is correct, but we need to review on-the-ground strategies so that all team members under-stand their roles, expectations, and the what-works for any given child. Gen-erally, when I think a child is ready to return to class, I wait a few minutes longer.

Those with a strong behavioral bent often critique this strategy. It is true that allowing a child to leave the classroom and have one-to-one time has the potential to reinforce the very act of leaving. The notion of a "push-in" strat-egy makes great sense when a child can be redirected. That is, staff support comes into the room rather than having the child transition to a different space. But if that child is fully dysregulated—or about to become that way—it is more effective to remove the child from the stimulation of the room, not to mention that it allows the child to save face in front of peers. And it enables the other students to continue learning, which is a core concern for any teacher. Being fully dysregulated is a state that no one would choose—many children and adults describe how draining and debilitating it feels—so it seems unlikely that attention from others would encourage such behavior. For a different set of children, especially those who tend toward mild, anxi-ety-driven task avoidance, being allowed to leave the room may well bolster the number of times such behavior occurs. As always, our interventions must be carefully geared to a specific child's needs and what works most effectively.

The notion of supporting children does not mean that we ignore the impact of the children's behaviors on others or even themselves. It is a ques-tion of timing, and the middle of a crisis is not when the doors are open to talk of consequences. Trauma is an explanation for many of the behaviors we see, but if we make it an excuse, we are heading down a very troubling road. Later, we will look at restitution, or restorative practice, as a productive way to address behavior.

If attempts to settle the child are not working, additional concrete steps should be clarified in the crisis intervention section of the support plan. Here are some of the questions that need to be answered:

1. At what point does the rest of the class need to be moved elsewhere if the child is not safe? Depending on the age of the students, who will help them transition out of the room? Where exactly will they go? This should be pre-determined if possible.

2. How long before someone contacts parents, the local crisis unit, or the police/ambulance, if necessary? If it is not a decision based on an amount of time, which specific behaviors rise to the level of asking for outside help?

3. Who will make the decision?

4. Who is responsible for making the necessary phone calls?

5. Who will stay with the child to make sure the child is safe?

6. Since one adult should not be alone with a dysregulated child, who will intervene to help stabilize an escalated situation?

7. What is the district policy regarding hands-on restraint? Have staff been properly trained? Are they certified?

8. Who will follow up with the other students who may have heard disturbing comments or seen upsetting behaviors? In crisis-speak, it is a question of who will debrief everyone, including, if necessary, classroom staff.

These are details that need to be resolved before landing in the middle of a crisis. Teachers and other staff—paraprofessionals, counselors, school nurses, and administrators—must be familiar with and, ideally, practiced in the details of the plan, which should reduce their own stress and allow them to address issues more confidently. Unfortunately, it is often this preparation phase that gets missed in schools because everyone is stretched for time, but it is time well spent. Rather than develop an intervention on the fly or replicate what is not working each time an issue suddenly arises, a collaborative planning process lets us fine-tune our set of approaches. The child study team or student adjustment team—schools call these planning meetings by various names—is the ideal setting for doing this kind of joint problem-solving work.

My preference is for children to know and understand their support plans just as they should understand the details of any behavior plan in place for them (see Levine, 2007). They must be given the opportunity to provide input into the plan as well. Children with trauma need to be able to predict to some extent what others will do and say; reviewing the plan in a meaningful way allows them to anticipate and feel more in control. It certainly does not mean that they will like the plan or appreciate having one, but it does remove the element of surprise. Not to mention, it is a respectful act and reflects that adults are committed to involving children in the process. When this is the prevailing attitude, there is usually less fight over control since the child has the opportunity to participate in a meaningful way. I have spoken with children who, later, recall few of the specifics of their support plans but remember how it felt to them to be included in the problem-solving and decision-making aspects.

To summarize, the support plan, the Basic Pyramid, is based on three overarching steps: (1) prevention, (2) redirection, and (3) crisis intervention. The following is a case example of how it works in practice.

Gerald is a white, 15-year-old 10th grader. To say he has a trauma history is an understatement. On the ACEs scale, he is a 10 out of 10; he likes to joke, "I have a perfect score." Until his trauma was formally diagnosed, he carried a stew of different mental health diagnoses. Without delving too far into the sad and disturbing details of his life, it is not a stretch to say that he has experienced more trauma than most. His father, severely alcoholic, was killed in a drunk-driving accident; Gerald was in the car but escaped with only a few broken bones. This was when he was six. His mother has had a long history of mental illness and addiction. She was badly beaten by a man she had been seeing after her husband's fatal accident; Gerald was barely nine at the time. Since then he has lived with a step-grandparent, who took him in but was not enthralled about "having to do it." Despite this history, Gerald is a boy with a sly sense of humor, someone who easily grasps the subtleties of conversation and other people's humor, and has a strong, almost fierce intelligence. I liked him immediately. He is also struggling in school, especially in reading and writing, and this causes him embarrassment and no small amount of anger. He has outbursts in class, is described as "combustible" by some of his teachers, and scares his classmates, even though he can be kind and engaging. Other students thought he was funny at first, but the ferocity of his outbursts led them to keep their distance. In addition, he is a self-described "control fiend," which has led to confrontations with both adults and peers.

Fortunately, Gerald is willing to talk about his behavior, something many adolescents his age passionately avoid. (This is whether they have trauma or not.) He knows that his behaviors bring him the exact opposite of what he wants, which is more friends and less conflict. He finally started seeing a therapist six months ago, which he first found confusing and "hard," but over time he began to feel more comfortable with his sessions. It took repeated attempts, but his step-grandparent was finally persuaded to follow through on therapy by the school's principal, who stepped in to push the issue. Because there was no feasible way for Gerald to get to appointments, he began seeing someone who was already coming into the school from a local community mental health agency.

In speaking with this therapist (I was consultant to Gerald's school), it was clear that talking about his family history was not helpful to Gerald. It tended to land him in an angry, almost dissociative funk. So they switched their focus to dealing with current issues and ways to self-regulate. For him, a combination of old-fashioned isometric exercises—for example, pushing his palms together as hard as he could and repeating the process multiple times—and then taking deep breaths seemed helpful, at least some of the time. This was progress, since Gerald previously had no strategies to pull from other than to bolt from the room. When he was younger, he simply hit people.

In school, we brainstormed other strategies, some of which he found helpful and others not at all. For example, taking a fast walk in the hallway was sometimes beneficial. He had a prescribed route so that staff would know where he was. Sitting in a small, contained space in the sensory room— almost the very opposite of his general tendency to seek out open spaces where he could run—worked well for him at times, especially if he could squeeze a stress ball with full force. (He literally destroyed a full set of these balls.) Gerald also did hundreds of chair push-ups in that space, a sensory intervention he figured out on his own. Finally, he developed an attachment to one of the special-education teachers in the building, and she allowed him to spend time sitting quietly in her classroom if he needed to. It was interesting that he could stay quiet in that room but not in other settings; clearly, she was an anchor for him. The goal, of course, was to help him reach the point where he could use strategies within his own classroom rather than having to leave, but that was a longer-term goal.

A side note: Someone more strictly behavioral in their approach would suggest that the last option above should *not* have been made available to Gerald. I can anticipate the question: Won't sitting with a favorite teacher reinforce his acting in ways that allow him to do this more often? The answer is an emphatic no. Because Gerald cared deeply about not "bothering other people" and was ashamed of those times he lost control, he did not seek out this teacher when he was struggling. Typically, it needed to be offered to him as an option. Sometimes he made use of it; sometimes he did not. An outcome like this points to why we need to understand a child and the impact of trauma rather than lean too heavily on a single clinical perspective.

As noted earlier, redirection is the critical step often given less attention than it deserves. Gerald preferred a quiet reminder that he was "getting there," meaning that he was heading toward a crisis. People would try cuing him to take a quick walk or get some water, which worked some of the time but not all the time. These are not new strategies, but fitting them into a larger framework and categorizing them in the language of redirection was novel for everyone involved, including Gerald. Another redirective approach was to quietly tell him that the teacher would help him through a task and that he did not need to do it on his own if he was becoming overwhelmed. In other words, the emphasis on student "independence" went out the window at times like these. Teachers used these reminders in a joining way rather than as threats or a message of rejection, and once Gerald perceived them as they were intended, he could accept that he needed to try them. And these simple strategies made a difference, as Gerald slowly began to have fewer full-blown crises. Redirection is not a complicated concept, but the steps need to be well-defined—or "operationalized"—and the entire process rooted in supportive relationships with adults who (in Gerald's words) "get it."

There is no manual for how to redirect children who are about to go past their threshold for coping. Whatever strategies are in place, I have rarely seen success unless the children understands *why* it is being suggested that they get some water, take a break, pull out their paper for journaling or coloring, visualize a peaceful setting, and so forth. In addition, anything that removes the focus on what is wrong in the moment can serve as a form of redirection; the artistry lies in applying it with the right timing, tone, and message. Those of us in the field all know adults who seem to manage well in these charged situations and others who struggle with them. Some of this, of course, is due to the adult's own temperament, history, experience, and ability to connect with traumatized and sometimes challenging children. Gerald was in the right environment for his needs: with adults who were willing to work diligently at it. They asked many questions, discussed things among themselves, and made a genuine commitment to help this young man.

The approach to crisis intervention for Gerald was based on a finite number of steps. Continuing to focus on de-escalation was paramount. In a few highly escalated instances, he was able to recount that he did not fully take in the words people had to say but that he could make sense of the tone of voice. He intuitively recognized an offer of support in comparison to the alternative—threats, stern lecturing, and mentions of punishment—and, according to him, it made a significant difference. The school counselor was called in on some occasions to help him settle down, which generally worked successfully except in one notable instance: Gerald became so disorganized and upset, punching himself in the head with his fists and talking so loudly that, while other students were being removed from the room, the school contacted the area crisis unit. Upon hearing the story, the crisis clinician had an ambulance sent in. Gerald was hospitalized for three days and then spent almost two weeks in a partial hospitalization program. As in many districts, there was a reentry meeting when Gerald was ready to return to school, where the support plan was again reviewed. Fortunately, that has been the only event of this magnitude and, overall, Gerald is stable, spending more time in class, and making reasonable academic progress. Recently, I saw a young man whose mood was brighter, who was more engaged in class and significantly less edgy and socially isolated.

Here, in summary, are the Pyramid steps for supporting Gerald in the classroom:

Prevention:

1. Wean Gerald off an existing behavior plan. It focuses on "earning" and "not earning" points with the stated goals of "act respectfully" and "complete your academic work." The plan creates stress and anger for him; it is not helping him to learn new self-regulation skills, the lack of which are the

underlying reason for many of his presenting behavioral problems. In addition, the plan has been used only intermittently and for a long period of time. This suggests the plan itself is no longer implanted with fidelity.

2. Remind him, if necessary, to use his isometric-type exercises followed by deep breaths.

3. Have him take a fast-paced walk in a known location where he can be monitored.

4. Suggest he visit the occupational therapy sensory room if there is not another student in that space.

5. Offer him the opportunity to sit quietly in the special-education teacher's room. (She has not had a problem with his behavior even once. Notably, this option has not increased his leaving from his scheduled classes.)

6. Remind him to use his self-calming strategies. Name them if necessary.

7. As part of the team discussion, consider what we know and do not know about Gerald's triggers. That is, what situations or people are most likely to set him off? He does not feel comfortable with one of his teachers in particular; he is morbidly uncomfortable with being called on in class; and he wants to be praised privately for positive effort rather than in front of his classmates.

8. Consider the best ways to connect with Gerald on a personal level. What works and what does not? What are the most effective ways to talk with him?

9. Brainstorm about restitution and ways Gerald can make it up to others.

10. Consider his academic areas of strength and need. Review conclusions from the RTI process, and make sure that these recommendations are being implemented.

11. Maintain ongoing collaboration with Gerald's primary care physician and outside therapist. Send short summaries of his behavior to the prescriber. This last step is made more important by the fact that his guardian is not a reliable reporter, nor does she check in with the school to see how he is doing.

Redirection:

1. Ask Gerald to go to the water fountain to get a drink. Remind him he can take a walk if necessary. Similarly, ask him to "get something from the office" if this will help him focus his energies (and if he is not yet too escalated).

2. Remind him to use any self-calming strategies that he has available. (I use this strategy across all three phases of the Pyramid.) If necessary, he can keep a small written list of them in case he is too agitated to remember the strategies.

3.   Make a quiet offer to help him rather than push him to take on an academic task independently.

4.   Use a calm voice, as few words as possible, and a nonthreatening stance.

5.   Act quickly upon seeing Gerald starting to clench, grimace, and/or start talking loudly, since he usually will continue to escalate without intervention. Ignoring is not a successful strategy.

Crisis intervention:

1.   Continue trying to de-escalate him by staying quietly in sight but not necessarily speaking with him at first. Ask him if he is "ready to talk" before proceeding.

2.   Once again, remind him to use his self-calming strategies. State them explicitly if he cannot remember or access them. Ask first if he is ready to hear them.

3.   Avoid direct eye contact or staring at him.

4.   Ask other students to leave if needed, usually at the point at which Gerald's voice is becoming increasingly loud and his fists are clenched.

5.   Require the teacher to call the office for someone to join her in the classroom. If Gerald becomes physically aggressive, such as attempting to break things, the school will wait up to 20 minutes to see if he can begin to show signs of de-escalation. If not, or if his behavior builds to where it becomes a safety risk to himself or others, the school will call the guardian and their local crisis team. If there is not a timely response, they will immediately call the local police.

There should be careful consideration as to how often children need to review the elements of the plan with one or more members of their team. Some children require at least twice-daily check-ins, at least to start. In schools with a "check-in, check-out" program, this fits perfectly into existing planning. No matter how it is scheduled into a child's day, I prefer short, frequent check-ins, especially at the start, because many children with PTSD cannot tolerate longer verbal exchanges or a too-intense self-reflection process. Gerald was scheduled in exactly such a way. In addition, in the short term, some children need a check-in during the *middle* of the day (which was not the scenario for Gerald). This is where a careful approach to planning is necessary. While it sounds time-intensive, these meetings are brief, often not more than two minutes or so. Knowing he could anticipate these calming moments mattered a great deal to Gerald; that was something he was able to articulate clearly.

Feedback does not need to be provided by a school counselor. Some have overwhelming caseloads and are called upon to do extensive crisis intervention as well as attend all kinds of meetings. Any adult can take on the role, but with guidance from the counselor and regular opportunities to ask questions and review how the process is working. Again, this is not therapy; it is a focused, skills-building review. The most significant aspect is that any student, including Gerald, can depend on it. It is equally important that the child understands the process for what it is, a teaching and learning scenario rather than a crucible of negative judgment.

Some children respond best when one person takes over the reins for doing these reviews. Given some children's lack of trust, many can build such trust with only one adult at a time. It is too intrusive—and the bar is set too high—when they are suddenly expected to connect with multiple adults all at once. This, of course, depends on the children, the nature of their relationships, the degree of trauma and the level of trust with which they individually come to us. The point is to assess these factors when determining who should check in with a given child and thinking through what the review process should look like. The process may sound complicated, but, in fact, it is not. It is a matter of planning, coordination, and attention to these kinds of details, although admittedly easier said than done when everyone is scrambling for time.

Along with the three phases of the support plan, it is important to note *when* a follow-up meeting of support team members will take place. This piece is often missing. Otherwise, it may take an additional crisis before people return to the table. A support plan created with little to no formal follow-up leads to not only an ineffectual plan but, even more seriously, a child who may not be able to trust that adults will follow through on their commitments. I observed a child who was "pissed off" and said, in effect, that he did not care so much if the plan was working right then but wanted someone to talk with him about it and where things were headed. Such commentary is instructive if we listen closely to its message.

In isolation, the steps in Gerald's support plan are not complicated. Putting them in a logical sequence and ensuring that they were both detailed and clearly understood by all pertinent staff—and, significantly, by Gerald—contributed to improvements in his behavior. For each child the model is applied differently, but the larger concepts are the same. Anyone looking at the support plan should be able to quickly and easily grasp the basic approach and set of strategies. The details, however, require the team to take the time to sit down at the table and discuss. In the more challenging situations, it helps to "drill" or rehearse the different interventions, typically through role play. De-escalation during a crisis, for example, is rarely simple. This skill alone takes practice unless one has had previous experience. And it is done differently depending on the child and the situation at hand.

In contrast to how we typically approach setting up our interventions, a "logical sequence" may mean something entirely different for each child when it comes to the Pyramid. For some children, starting with the crisis response is needed; they want to know what will happen during the most distressing episodes. There is no formula for when to begin with this stage. Sometimes, I have simply asked children, "Where do you want to start?" after showing them and describing what the model looks like. In these situations, children who have experienced the most severe forms of abuse may want to know, from their perspective, what the worst is that we can throw at them. Many are relieved to learn that this is a collaborative process with a nonpunishing orientation. One boy told me he was literally "shocked" that the Pyramid is intended only to help him. After years of failing—his term— on different incentive plans, which generated a great deal of anger and resentment, it took him a little while to grasp (and to hold onto the idea) that the Pyramid was meant to support him. He also needed to know, more than once, that the plan was not oriented to "taking things away" from him. That statement alone tells us how he perceived incentive-based behavior plans.

A benefit of the Pyramid's format lies in its simplicity, and at the same time, it reminds us to focus holistically on the child rather than on narrow areas of intervention. I find that for children who are regularly in crisis, there is less discussion about prevention and redirection; the focus, understandably, is what to do when a crisis erupts. But those interventions related to prevention and redirection are what generally contribute to reducing the number—and severity—of crisis situations. However, if the child has not recently experienced a serious incident, there is a tendency to forget about the content in the crisis section of the plan, and therefore, if a crisis erupts suddenly, people may be unprepared. Maintaining some level of attention to each of the three sections of the support plan is critical, especially for the most involved and complex children with trauma.

Another component of good planning is determining the relevant outside services a child needs. Whether it is to reach out to the child's primary care physician, help arrange individual or family therapy (or both), assist in facilitating a referral to a prescriber, or coordinate a different service, the school counselor can adopt a case management role so that there is appropriate outreach and communication. Getting releases signed by parents or guardians is part of this, something generally simple to accomplish unless there is a problematic relationship between school and home.

Finally, staff self-reflection is a crucial piece if the Pyramid is to be used most effectively. Teachers, counselors, administrators—and caregivers, too—are virtually always struggling to keep up, meaning the time needs to be carved out from somewhere else in their day. I find that the faster I run to try to keep up, the more I resort to doing more of what I already know—or think I know. The value in engaging in self-reflection has been demonstrated across professional fields. Schön (1983) was an early proponent and wrote what is still a classic text in the field. Hall and Simeral (2008) later added to the literature, focusing exclusively on educators. They quote John Dewey's famous comment: "It's not the doing that matters; it's the thinking about the doing." In other words, the Pyramid's preplanning process, our considerations about what does and does not work, our brainstorming about other creative ways to help a child if the process is not bringing substantive improvement—all of these are working examples of reflection in action. These are much needed steps, especially when trying to intervene with some of our most complicated and distressed children.

CHAPTER THREE

Differences between the Basic Pyramid and Traditional Behavior Plans

Many teachers and parents report that the language tied to what we refer to as behavior plans is confusing. For me, behavior plans—or as they are formally called in schools, "behavior intervention plans (BIPs)"—signify that there are incentives attached to specific behaviors or skills we are attempting to teach/shape. The child will earn (or not earn) rewards based on whether the targeted behavior meets an established goal. This kind of plan differs from a support plan (the Pyramid falls under this other category), a safety plan, a crisis plan, or any of the other names given to these various and overlapping interventions. A behavior plan can be used as part of these other plans, but it is a distinct intervention based on increasing specific behaviors and reducing unwanted ones. While this may sound rather simplistic, I find that the terms are used interchangeably to the point where there is little consensus about what they mean and what they are intended to do. I know experienced counselors and principals who report that they continue to stumble over the different terminology.

Another difference lies in how these plans are sequenced. Behavior plans are typically reactive; that is, they are put in place because a child's behavior has become disruptive—or, in the words of one caregiver, "bothersome"—in some way. They come into being *after* problems have arisen. In contrast, the Pyramid can be used *before* any kind of behavior problem presents itself. These interventions can be generated because of behavioral issues, but they can also be implemented because a child is sad, anxious, and struggling overall. If a behavior plan is used as part of the support plan, I locate it in the "Prevention" section. This is where it is best understood as a teaching tool rather than as a consequence for whatever negative behaviors the child displays.

I infrequently use behavior plans with children who have known or suspected trauma histories. There are exceptions, especially for children also exhibiting signs of ADHD who need short-term incentives to help them focus or learn new strategies, but these are not the norm. When I do believe a formal behavior plan is needed, I use the model outlined in my earlier book, *Learning from Behavior* (initially published in 2007). This is a relationally based model, meaning that while there are incentives attached to the plan, the approach is supportive, feedback-oriented, and positive. It relies on the idea that the quality of children's relationships counts as much if not more than the specific tool we employ to support change.

This strategy of using limited behavior plans seems to go against the grain for many clinicians, teachers, and parents as well as administrators in school systems, juvenile justice settings, and the like. Why adopt this position? The reason is that, even when behavior plans are applied carefully and with much thought, children often find the plans coercive and symbolic of their loss of control; this, of course, is the opposite of what we are trying to achieve. And for those children with poor frustration tolerance, or what one boy ruefully calls his "extremely short fuse that gets loud when it blows," a minor not-earn on a reward plan can ignite a full-blown rage or shut down. These are meant as *teaching* tools, and it is critical to make sure that they are implemented from this clinical and philosophical perspective. For some children, we cannot achieve this. That is, no matter how skillfully—and sensitively—we use these plans, they may still represent reward-and-punishment thinking rather than meaningful attempts to build new skills. Typically, I find that children experience them as a judgment about their goodness and worth, which is not a helpful perspective for any child and especially not those with trauma.

In one way or another, I have been involved in hundreds of behavior plans. While there have been success stories, more often I see traumatized children's frustration, powerlessness, and anger. Teachers and caregivers often find them hard to implement, especially in terms of maintaining consistency—*fidelity*, as the term is now used in schools—and providing the necessary feedback. Failure on a behavior plan can leave a traumatized child literally seething with bitterness and resentment. I have observed children with an increasing sense of learned helplessness, a hallmark of depression, when they cannot succeed. In short, they give up and stop trying. Again, these interventions have a place in our toolkits, but they should be complementary rather than primary interventions. Among children with trauma, I have seen many more negatives than positives.

In contrast to behavior plans, the Pyramid is a continuum-of-care model and intended primarily to help children learn to cope with trauma. The goal is to clarify interventions whether there are (1) no current issues, (2) early signs of trouble, or (3) a full-blown crisis. It aims to give children more control and predictability by focusing on building self-calming skills and ways to manage. There are no rewards attached to specific behaviors, so children cannot "fail" on the plan. The Pyramid, then, is oriented very differently from a traditional behavior plan. It reflects a global approach that clarifies and provides a structured intervention: thus its description as a *support plan*.

The Pyramid should be *in addition* to whole-school interventions for helping all students. This is not an either/or situation. In RTI language, part of the MTSS model that is now widespread in schools, a Tier 1 approach to making every child feel welcome, known, and less stressed will bring benefits across the board. We know that large numbers of children come to school—or go home to a caregiver—carrying the burdens of their traumatic experiences. Therefore, many schools and districts have adopted trauma-informed approaches on a universal basis, whether as part of their instructional methods or by setting up calming corners in each classroom. The Pyramid, in comparison, is specific to individual children who need more intensive, individualized care, meaning it is a Tier 3 approach. It is the same within caregivers' settings; using a structured intervention may be necessary, but this does not preclude looking at the larger home environment and how it contributes to—or derails—a child's well-being and sense of safety.

How We Can Talk with Children about the Basic Pyramid

It is expected somehow that teachers, other school staff, and caregivers instinctively know how to broach a discussion of using a support plan, or any other kind of intervention, with children. My experience is that this is anything but the case. As in addressing any other sensitive topic, some adults are more comfortable with this than others. I have heard from many people that they want to help; they want to be involved and participate in implementing strategies that make sense. But, as they admit, it is anxiety-provoking to think about having the actual discussion with children. Questions I hear: How do I communicate what needs to be said? Will I cause the child to become upset? Will the child blow up and run away or become aggressive? Will I make things worse? What will happen if *I* get angry if the child is defiant and unwilling to engage? And notably, some people worry that children will resent and even "hate" them for raising the subject. I can understand such worries, as holding these kinds of conversations is not something that comes automatically or easily to many of us. It is a harmful myth that, as adults, we should always know the "right" things to say. By "harmful," I mean that this implicit expectation may in turn keep us from asking necessary questions, learning more about what we ought to know, and delving into the very conversations children need to have.

Shea (2017) offers a helpful framework for thinking more deeply about this process. Since one major focus of his clinical work is to elicit any hidden suicidal thinking among his patients, it seems evident that he would therefore need to carefully consider what he refers to as the "art of the interview." As a psychiatrist, his is a psychological slant, but his strategies are relevant to virtually anyone in the helping professions who is put in the position of having these types of difficult conversations.

Shea introduces ideas that are especially relevant to how to converse with traumatized children about using the Pyramid. One is the notion of what he calls "shame attenuation." We will be discussing the role of shame in the next chapter. For now, however, it is worth noting this concept in the context of how we introduce the model. In short, Shea looks to make his adult patients less intimidated and, as a result, less defensive. So in describing the Pyramid to a child, we might say something like, "With everything you've been going through, we thought it might help to try. . . ." In other words, the goal is to reduce any possible stigma that the child might assume is linked to having a support plan in place.

Another of Shea's strategies is what he refers to as "normalization." He emphasizes this as an interviewing technique, stating clearly that anyone in this person's position would need some type of assistance. It is a subtle but powerful way of framing language that can be adapted for talking with children about the Pyramid. When a child has a sense of having been forcefully "put" on a plan—any kind of plan—and comes to the table already feeling one-down, it takes some dedicated rapport-building and attention to using sensitive language to reach a kind of buy-in. I have been struck at times by how the dialogue—if there is actually any real back-and-forth at all—can be strident, one-sided, and representative of almost the opposite of normalization. Instead, it may come across as though there is something deeply wrong with the child, that the adults are angry and thus we need to, as one irate boy told me, "shove it down [his] . . . throat." It is true that the child needs a support plan, but we also want the child to be willing to participate. *How* we put it on the table for discussion requires thoughtful consideration, just as we need to carefully think through the *what* of the plan.

It is not only about a child's anger. Combating hopelessness is equally critical. We know that hopelessness is a primary component of suicide, whether in thoughts or actions. This state can be situational or a general attitude toward life. For children with PTSD, it is usually more the latter and thus harder to confront. As a result, any intervention has to rest on a realistic sense of optimism and positive belief. By communicating the critical message that we will provide a structure, a form of safety that also promotes greater optimism, we have a vastly better chance of enlisting the child's willingness to participate and, hopefully, the child's own capacity to believe that things can improve.

Shea contends that some degree of letting go of bitterness for the past, no matter how severe one's trauma, and developing more confidence in the future is the recipe for creating better problem-solving skills. Drawing from his ideas, this would allow a child to live more in the present moment, that is, with empathy and even with some degree of humor. Without those conditions, living in the present is much less possible. All this translates back to the idea that the Pyramid is more than a technical tool of the trade. How it is introduced, worded, implemented, and reviewed is critical if we are to help the child begin to move away from a state of hopelessness and shift toward using better problem-solving skills. The process matters.

Taking this a step further, Shea points to the "science of empathy." His focus is something called facilics, which, in short, refers to structuring an interview so that it feels more like an "engaging" conversation rather than a scripted question-and-answer session. Although he presents this concept in the context of talking with people about their suicidal thoughts and plans, it is equally pertinent to our conversations with traumatized children about their behavior and ways of coping. I have witnessed initial discussions of interventions that come across as caring and genuine; I have also sometimes observed them when these discussions communicate disappointment, frustration, and the underlying message, "I don't know what else to do with you." If reducing hopelessness is a primary goal, the latter clearly will not help. To state the obvious, most educators and caregivers do not go into these discussions attempting to make children feel worse, but it does happen. It takes reflection and a willingness to think about the process *first* that will help reduce these outcomes.

Riess (2017), a physician who studies patient satisfaction in health care, dives further into the discussion about empathy, which she describes as both a learnable skill—it is not "hardwired," as had been presumed some years ago—and closely linked with compassion. She says, "A cardinal feature of empathy is that it usually helps connect people to others" (p. 75); it is a simple and straightforward statement, one that adheres perfectly with the notion that by demonstrating empathy when we talk with children about using the Pyramid, there is likely to be greater investment in and more agreement over moving forward with this intervention. As such, Riess—as well as Medina (Johnson, 2019), a developmental molecular biologist who studies the human brain and created what he calls "brain rules"—shows us that empathy can contribute to strategic progress. It takes us beyond the fuzzy cultural prescription simply to be nice to children.

Norcross and Wampold (2019), two psychologists who rigorously study what works—and what does not—in psychotherapy, stress that the quality of the relationship in the room is more important than any specific therapeutic technique. They do not disparage the significance of method, but the strength of the relationship—the words *attunement* and *empathy* are often applied in this context—is seen as paramount. Again, this filters into the discussion with a child about how the Pyramid can be used to help. It reminds us yet again that the nature of the conversation with that child is what drives whether the child is likely to accept going forward with it or not.

Another factor to consider in terms of empathy is the congruence of facial expressions, tone, and message when talking with children about challenging topics. Since children with PTSD are hypervigilant and continually watching to see that they are safe, many will quickly perceive when these different forms of communication do not match. One clinician, who works with challenging children and their caregivers, told me a story about a child who challenged him directly on how he delivered a message about an impending hospitalization. This clinician, smart, self-reflective, and a role model for younger clinicians, grimaced as he remembered this scenario. In that instance, he smiled gently at the child in the attempt, he said, to "soften the message." That was not how it was received. In therapy terms, it was an empathic failure. The child was infuriated not only about an involuntary hospitalization but also by the fact that, in his perception, the clinician thought this was something worth smiling about. A lesson not forgotten, I was told. When we talk with children about the Pyramid, therefore, we need to be mindful of our own way of communicating during the process. This is an interactive dialogue, not just a listening event for the child. Our own self-awareness is a main factor in whether the Pyramid has any chance to result in a successful outcome.

It helps to be an attentive observer. One child with a history of sexual abuse reported that her abuser used to "smile at her" before and after each incident. This is both chilling and not uncommon. She therefore learned not to trust adults smiling at her, especially if she perceived that their eyes were not smiling in concert with the rest of their face. Knowing this piece of her history, and observing carefully during any discussion of the Pyramid, helped the process immeasurably. We may never have known—it was a fortunate bit of good collaboration in this case—but anyone carefully observing this girl would be able to see how she recoiled when adults, with their eyes aimed directly at her face, smiled broadly.

Medina (Johnson, 2019) argues that empathic teachers generate higher test scores among their students. I do not know that there is hard data to back such an assertion, but the idea certainly resonates with me. If empathy and thus connection mean more safety for a traumatized child, it frees up mental space for learning. By extension, having these factors in place would suggest that a child with PTSD could focus less on safety and more on growth.

This has been a great deal of discussion about the subject of empathy. But given the demands of contemporary students and the state of our current approaches, we need to advance both the complexity of our thinking and the precision of our interventions.

Another consideration for how to broach the subject of using the Pyramid is related to children's motivation. Along with whether a child trusts that this could be a helpful rather than harmful tool, it also matters if this child believes there is reason to want to change. I have listened to many stories about how everyone should "treat me better" or "just leave me alone" and not heard a willingness to look inward and think about how to cope more effectively. It may certainly be true that others have historically been unkind, but children still need to develop critical self-regulation skills so they can manage in the present.

Given this, *Motivational Interviewing* (MI), by Miller and Rollnick (2013) is applicable. The model, which emerged from the authors' work in the field of substance abuse and was first developed for work with adults, argues for the effectiveness of joint goal setting rather than confrontation. Miller and Rollnick advocate for the idea that by supporting people to articulate and establish their own goals, their current behavior can then be compared directly to those personal goals. They developed the notion of "change talk," which frames the discussion away from a focus on problematic behavior and redirects it toward how to reach one's own goals. The model's concepts can easily be adapted to thinking about how to help children with PTSD. This is where the Pyramid comes in, as a tool to support that process of change.

In summary, this chapter not only provides an outline of how the model differs from traditional behavior plans but also offers various ideas for how to introduce and implement it. The structure of the Pyramid is relatively simple; how we engage and talk with children and then implement it on a relational level are factors worth our continued reflection as well as additional scientific study.

CHAPTER FOUR

The Impact of Shame

After looking at how the Pyramid works both in practice and in its approach to communication, let's continue the discussion about trauma and, in formal diagnostic terms, PTSD. While having in place a specific, well-defined support plan such as the Pyramid is essential, deepening our understanding of additional factors related to trauma will only improve our work and help us at every phase of intervention.

Shame is a primary emotional underpinning of trauma—not necessarily all forms of trauma but especially those related to sexual, physical, and emotional abuse as well as to witnessing domestic violence. It can also be the result of repeated bullying, a term not used lightly here, or insidious if not overt forms of racism as well as other types of discrimination and bigotry.

It is worth remembering that younger children may engage in magical thinking, meaning they believe that if they had only done things differently, there would have been a better outcome. This arises in the context of tornadoes, floods, and other kinds of natural disasters. One boy, approximately seven years old, told me that if he had only "behaved," there would not have been the fire that burned down his house. (It was due to an electrical fire.) Self-blame and shame can gnaw at us at any age.

The usual distinction between shame and guilt is that the latter involves our behavior—something we did—and the former is a more deeply embedded vision of how we view ourselves: in essence, the very root of our being. I hear the sentences "I'm bad," "There's something wrong with me," "No one really cares what happens to me," and "My life is out of control" more times than I can quantify. These statements reflect what shame can do to a child's inner dialogue and meaning making.

Shame is defined as a "painful feeling that's a mix of regret, self-hate, and dishonor" (https://www.vocabulary.com/dictionary/shame). Coles (2000) refers to the harmful impact of what he calls "tenacious despair." The word "falseness" also gets mention, which I think is both apt and powerful. Children with trauma consistently report feeling as though they cannot maintain a strong or consistent vision of who they are, which impedes their developing a coherent identity. Adults may describe an almost permanent sense of being "adrift" or "fragmented." Psychoanalytic thinkers describe the "false self," an idea first introduced by Winnicott (1960), to explain the protective front meant to guard against one's shame and stress. Different kinds of personas arise as a result: for example, the "tough guy," or "the helper" who will go beyond all reasonable lengths to assist others. This all translates to the idea that traumatized children often have a poorly developed sense of self, leaving them confused—and overflowing with shame. The question "Who am I?" is a normal part of development, but it is magnified many times over among these children.

According to Burgo (2018), there are four subtypes of shame: (1) unrequited love, which, in short, represents rejection; (2) unwanted exposure, such as getting called out in front of an entire class for doing something wrong or when others see you doing something you wish they hadn't (which, says Burgo, is the type that typically comes to mind when one hears the word *shame*); (3) disappointed expectation, which is self-explanatory—a child feels hurt for not getting what the child wanted or anticipated, such as a visit from a noncustodial parent; and (4) exclusion, which refers to being (and feeling) left out. Burgo suggests that all people want desperately to fit in and belong, a simple idea that, when applied to traumatized children, might explain many of the behaviors we witness. In general, according to Kelly and Lamia (2018, introduction), "shame continually influences the way we care in our relationships."

Bradshaw (2005) identifies a different type—or perhaps more accurately, a different wording—that he refers to as "toxic shame." He indicates that that all forms of child sexual abuse, especially those involving incest, can cause particularly severe toxic shame. This type of shame is buried deep within a child, leading to what is known as "complex trauma." Toxic shame, when it emerges, forces a child to dissociate—to self-distance—until there is some way to cope with it. I have witnessed children in this kind of mental turmoil and it can only be described as watching someone in a state of shock. They are simply not present. The resulting dissociation makes sense as a way to survive in the moment, but it leaves children numb, distressed, and out of touch with others—and themselves.

Piaget (1936), whose well-known work significantly impacts the fields of both education and psychology, describes four stages of cognitive development: sensorimotor, preoperational, concrete operations, and formal operations. It is the first two that need consideration here. *Sensorimotor* development is essentially just that: a child, through movement rather than language, explores and acts on immediate and direct stimuli in the child's environment. There is virtually no thinking process attached to this stage; instead, it is instinctive, reflexive, and fundamental to human life. Piaget saw this stage generally occurring between the ages of birth and two years, but he clarified that his stages were anything but "fixed" by a child's chronology. In other words, he looked at children developmentally—their "states"—rather than in terms of fixed "traits." During severe dissociation, whether it is activated by extreme shame or intrusive thoughts and memories, you can watch someone regress to this kind of developmental level in which no mental processing appears to take place. It represents distress, not intentional behavior, and trying to prod someone to think logically and prospectively during this period only causes additional stress. We understand this in practice, but Piaget's work offers a theoretical framework in support of these ideas.

Memorably, I once watched a 40-year-old woman with typical intelligence and a horrific trauma history regress to the point where she was literally crawling on the floor. Her use of language was not even in the form of words; instead, she uttered vocal sounds of discomfort and pointed to the too-bright lights in the waiting room. When, a little later, she was able to string together some short verbalizations, she repeated over and over that the room's low-level sounds were "hurting her ears." The same thing can happen with children when they are under severe stress. This is a living example of someone functioning at a sensorimotor level, an almost primitive way of interacting with one's surroundings. This same woman told me afterward that she had no recollection of these behaviors; it was almost as if she later awoke from a bad dream.

Piaget's second stage, called *preoperational*, is seen as generally occurring between ages two and seven. Here, children are able to think about their experiences but only as representations of "actual" rather than symbolic events. There is little applied logic, meaning that the child focuses solely on one event at a time—and often only on one aspect of it—and cannot connect it to other circumstances in life. In the language of schools, it means no generalization takes place. Piaget stresses that this means the child lacks the capacity to consider an experience in broader terms and can only perceive it through a narrow, egocentric lens: how it affects that child in that moment rather than anyone else or how that child might have been affected differently at other times. (Or how the child might have handled things differently in those other instances.) There is virtually no context or larger perspective at this stage of cognitive maturity, nor is there any real capacity for inferential thinking. In formal terms, Piaget refers to this kind of thinking as *centration*.

Therefore, a child who has regressed to this point due to some sort of activation of shame/trauma (or if this is the child's general level of functioning) will have very little ability in that moment to think things through calmly or rationally. Nor is the child likely to consider the impact on others. Educators often talk about the importance of *metacognition* in an academic context—how to think about what one knows and has learned—and that same principle applies to the emotional realm. Simply, it is not present during high-stress moments, so such actions as reflecting, considering consequences, and using problem-solving skills are not primary options; the "What's wrong" or "What happened" questions are essentially destined to fail. Instead, calming the child is paramount. Sometimes a simple, quiet "I can see you are upset, let's find a quiet place just to sit" comment is most effective.

Piaget's theory supports the idea that, in practice, when children regress due to their life experiences and resulting stress, there are times when they are *unable* to process events. We often look at these children and are astounded that bright, capable children are so incapacitated in these moments. Sometimes the only assumption that makes sense to us in the moment is that they are doing it intentionally or "looking for attention." It is usually anything but the case.

This does not necessarily exonerate the child, but there is a very real question about *when* the right time is to sit and explore what happened. And this reflects the underlying purpose as to why adults need to understand the three sections of the Basic Pyramid, which can help guide what to do (and when) based on thinking developmentally. For children with trauma, abilities during high-stress times are often in flux. At times, you can literally observe their coping skills appear and then suddenly disappear. We have to help them—and ourselves—prepare for this state of chaotic change.

A child with a long history (and early diagnosis) of PTSD told me that, under acute stress, she "forgets everything" she can do to help herself. She now carries a small notepad, which contains her own handwritten reminders along with some pictures she drew, so that she can read over her helping strategies when needed. For years, she was perceived as a child making willful choices to ignore both peers and the various adults in her life; only later did she discover and then share with significant others that this was not intentional but a way to cope with an onslaught of strong and chaotic emotions she could not comprehend or manage. Problem-solving was not available to her during these moments, nor could she make use of people trying to talk her through these raging feelings. This was a real-life combination of Piaget's theory and psychological regression in action. In simple terms, her thinking became disorganized and her behavior more erratic even though she was exceptionally bright and capable at other times.

There is a sizable body of literature on shame, both in and outside of discussions of trauma. (For more on the former, see van der Kolk, 2014 or Fisher, 2017.) We understand how shame can emerge. We also realize how a traumatized individual might self-medicate with alcohol and drugs in the attempt to numb overwhelming pain related both to the trauma and to those feelings of shame. If children experience physical or sexual abuse, we recognize that the children might conclude—mistakenly—that they did something wrong or were responsible for what happened. I met with a 17-year-old boy, a straight A student and excellent athlete, who drank and cut himself throughout his adolescence because he had absorbed the idea—carefully and maliciously promoted by his perpetrator—that he was to blame for his history of sexual abuse. When he could put words to his experience, the story he told about himself could only be defined as his holding deep-rooted feelings of shame. These were reflected in his vivid descriptions of disgust and self-blame. He described his internal dialogue as "always being in conflict with myself." This boy viewed events in the following way: It was all his fault; he caused it to happen; he is a defective person. As a result, he thought he needed to punish himself and deserved anything bad that happened to him.

This perspective is not uncommon among children who have been sexually or physically abused. I also discover it frequently in children who witness domestic violence at home and assume they should be able to put a hard stop to it. I hear this even from very young children, who believe that they are to blame when the reality is so clearly different. As one girl told me sadly, "Being ashamed really hurts your insides."

Shame, then, ties in with a sense of worthlessness and, in the words of the aforementioned 17-year-old boy, *badness*. The latter may not be a clinical term, but it is descriptive in ways that most clinical labels are not. To hold onto this vision, to have this belief worm its way into one's core, is what this same boy defined as "indescribably beyond painful." In his case, he internalized his pain instead of letting other people know or see it. But, inevitably, he couldn't contain such powerful feelings; they flooded out through a serious attempt at suicide. His words came later.

Shame is a profoundly internal experience, but it emerges through different emotions and behaviors: anger, aggression, depression, self-harm, anxiety . . . early substance use . . . addictions . . . a fundamental lack of belief in one's own competence. Given these potential difficulties and their overwhelming impact on a child's well-being, it is surprising that there has not been more dialogue about how shame ties in with childhood trauma.

An example is Terri, a white child of mixed ethnic background, who was abruptly told at the age of 10 that her birth was the result of her mother having been brutally raped. At the same time, she learned that her stepfather, whom she had always called "Dad," was not in fact her birth father. Shock does not adequately convey this child's reaction to discovering such painful information that, developmentally and emotionally, she was not ready to absorb. Her behavior changed sharply; her once-vibrant personality became subdued, darker, angrier. Her teachers had always described her in terms of the proverbial "sweet, happy, well-adjusted" child, but by the age of 12, those descriptors no longer applied. She was either distant and shut down or outwardly angry, disengaged from school and already experimenting with alcohol and marijuana. Alarmingly, she began showing signs of early sexual behavior, which was especially concerning to her parents, given her mother's history and their legitimate fear that Terri would not be able to keep herself safe. While many children's moods and behaviors begin to shift during their march into early adolescence, this was a rapid-fire change. After a serious cutting incident, she was hospitalized in an attempt to stabilize her and, more than a week later, she was referred to a partial hospitalization program.

Hospitalization did little to help Terri, at least according to her own report, but it was a short encounter with her school social worker there that began to change the tide. At this point Terri was 13 and completely floundering, and it was a surprise to her that anyone in school cared about her enough to come and visit her in the hospital. She was almost apologetic about the bland surroundings inside the unit. This school counselor did nothing more than express her wish that Terri start to feel better and it was enough to open the floodgates. She also repeatedly reminded Terri that she would be waiting for her in school when Terri returned. Terri, who had revealed almost nothing to the clinicians in the hospital and even less during group therapy sessions, expressed that she "really hated herself" and that she feared that every time her mother looked at her, she would be reminded of the horror of what had happened and how her daughter came to be born. She questioned whether her mother could love her as a result. Seeing herself in the mirror raised similar questions as to whether she could, in effect, ever love or even accept herself. She started to refer to herself, only half jokingly, as the bastard child. At one point, she had cut diagonal lines into her cheeks with a razor, typically a sign of distress if not outright dissociation. She expressed an alarming degree of self-disgust; her shame was evident. The possibility of her attempting suicide was never far from people's minds.

Whatever it was about the conversation with her school counselor that unlocked her in that specific moment led to a greater willingness to accept support. Sometimes it is a matter of timing or a familiar face and voice when they are most needed. It seems that the message of caring resonated for Terri in that place where, according to her, she felt "lonely, scared and all by myself." When she finally opened up to getting help, family therapy was necessarily an integral piece of the process.

The story is, of course, longer and more detailed but, in short, this is what shame can do to a child. While Terri may be seen as an extreme example, many traumatized and shame-filled children live with the belief that they are the cause of their families' unhappiness and discord. Sometimes they are given exactly that message. One boy told me that if he heard the words "if it wasn't for you" one more time, he would "hurt someone." This speaks to why it is imperative to help children with their misdirected belief systems—their interpretation of events and, thus, their meaning making—so that they can move on in healthier and more functional ways. It only complicates things and makes for a tougher climb out of despair when adults in a child's life perpetuate a blaming message. This happens more than we might wish, primarily so that adults can alleviate their own guilt and self-blame. One court-referred parent, accused of ongoing physical abuse, emphatically told me, "Clearly, it was [the child's] fault."

Tapping too quickly into individual children's humiliation, or worse, leaving children feeling wounded when they already carry a deep reservoir of shame, rarely contributes to a good outcome. This may sound obvious, but think about some of the statements you have heard. Maybe you yourself have slipped up in a highly charged or frustrating moment and said something you wish you had not; I think many of us have. Telling children with trauma that they "should be ashamed" of themselves, even when their behavior has been troubling, is highly unlikely to bring about a positive result. When shame is activated, it leads to a greater probability of aggression if not outright violence. I have seen serious outbursts by traumatized children when they perceive they are being put down or humiliated, even in situations when this was not the adult's intent. Eruptions can also arise unpredictably with peers in this same context. And when other children make an actual attempt to demean or bully them, the results can be dangerous, even tragic.

An example of this is the case of Theo, an African American, 12-year-old 6th grader, who was one of only two children of color in his entire grade—and the lone male. This was a suburban district with little diversity overall, but it was especially noticeable in his school. In addition, there were no staff who, he said, "looked like . . . [him]." His sense of isolation was compounded by the fact that his family had little money and that this was a relatively affluent district. Theo, two years earlier, had witnessed his father hit his mother during an argument and, to paraphrase his reporting of the incident, he felt paralyzed to do anything. In his mind, he knew he should call for help, but he became frozen to the spot. His younger sister called the police because "the yelling didn't stop." This, reportedly, was not the first time such an episode had occurred, but this one in particular stuck in Theo's mind, especially because two white police officers then came to arrest his father. The arrest, according to him, was handled roughly, and Theo told me he was furious with everyone—including himself because he "should have done something to help Mom and probably Dad too." At the same time, he acknowledged that he was embarrassed that it was his little sister who had to step up and call the police. He found himself thinking this at unexpected times, became ever more self-critical, and began to have occasional but intense nightmares.

His humiliation, the deeply ingrained belief that he was responsible for not protecting his mother, was poisonous for him. He became increasingly volatile, was defiant with teachers and got into some relatively small scrapes with other students, all of which were a change from how he had acted previously. Things exploded one day when two white teenagers teased him about a minor event at school. He described it to me later as the top of a volcano erupting from the internal buildup of pressure. He went after one of the boys, who initially was startled and reportedly tried to back away, but Theo could not stop himself. The other boy was older—and much bigger—and ended up breaking Theo's nose and eye socket. Even after getting hurt, he kept trying to fight. While Theo, in his own words, "lost the battle of fists," was injured, and got into serious trouble, I would describe him as almost relieved. He had, in his mind, stood up for himself, his family, and his race. He initially talked about how the incident was about "fighting against racism and oppression" but he came to believe that, while oppression is very real, those two boys were not trying to bully or humiliate him. Although he did not use these exact words, he was essentially reacting to shame. The two older boys had unwittingly tapped right into it. For Theo, it was a culmination of many different aspects of his life: his perception of being looked down on for being weak, Black, not rich, and the son of a man sent to prison.

I have known Theo for many years. He has grown from an angry 12-year-old into a thoughtful, reflective young man. He has never stepped away from calling out racism and other forms of bigotry, but he no longer uses his fists or "loses it." He is not ashamed but rightly angry when he senses unfairness. His father is now, as he puts it, "out of my life," although he would like to reestablish ties at some point. It took Theo a lot of work—and a willingness over time to talk openly with a white, male clinician, which did not come easily to him—to reduce his level of shame and the belief that he had failed his mother and, frankly, himself. As a result, he is now thoughtful, measured, and confident.

Admittedly, making a connection with Theo did not come easily for me either. He was smoldering with anger when I first met with him. He sized me up as "another white guy"—he told me this later—and did everything he could over the first few weeks to let me know that I did not and never would understand him. Clinicians within the therapeutic relationship, or the working alliance, describe a process known as *countertransference*, a psychoanalytic term still in use today. The process is defined by the clinician responding out of his own experience and, at the same time, reacting to the experience—and emotions—of the other person sitting across from him in the room. In this situation, I noted that he intensely disliked me before we even began and, for my part, I began to feel ashamed by not being able to reach him or help him in the least. Finally, one day, I told him this, and he softened dramatically. Therapy offers few real "aha" moments, but this was one of them, and the tide began to turn for both of us. Shame is a horrific feeling; we do all we can to deflect it.

In addition to aggressive behavior, overpowering shame can set off a dissociative state in which the person seems almost to disappear. Sitting with someone in this state is disorienting; it feels as though a curtain comes down and you are suddenly alone, even though the other person is physically right across from you. If one cannot tolerate the strength of this emotional shame, it is not hard to understand how such a phenomenon could occur. In the scientific language of neurology, becoming engulfed in shame leads to the amygdala taking over for—or hijacking—the frontal lobes, the thinking and planning portions of one's brain, leading to powerful reactions little associated with conscious thought. This means, as a result, there will be a reduced capacity to problem-solve or consider the implications of one's actions. In severe dissociation, these cognitive processes shut down.

In a clinic setting many years ago, I met with a young woman who, on the surface, appeared fine about describing her history of physical and sexual trauma. She was articulate, well-dressed, and seemingly calm. Moments later, she "disappeared" into herself—it is the only way I can describe it— and I had the frightening impression that no one else was in the room with me. Her eyes were vacant and staring straight ahead. She was completely shut down, her brain's response to telling a story she had long held inside and not shared due to her underlying belief that she had "caused" the problem. In other words, she experienced an intolerable onslaught of shame. Fortunately, because this was our fourth session together, I think she realized at some fundamental level that she was safe in the room with me and slowly came back into being present. Much later, she was able to put language to that experience and even joke about her "disappearing act."

Hallward (2014) refers to shame as a "lethal public health threat." She discusses shame's integral connection with depression and to the worthlessness and hopelessness linked to suicide. However, there is disagreement over whether children should be encouraged to "tell their stories." I do not believe that her conclusions about "traumatic silence" necessarily apply to everyone, especially children. In short, Hallward suggests that it is the silence itself that worsens shame. Staying quiet when quiet is imposed by an external source—a threatening adult, for example—is toxic. So is enforcement through an internal voice saying that one's secret story is too horrible to be put into words and named aloud. Nonetheless, even in a supportive environment, some children do not have the words to describe their experiences. In addition, we need to respect that every culture has its own ways of expressing grief and suffering. The idea of making space for one to tell one's story is vital, but pushing someone to do so is not. I have, unfortunately, seen this happen. In psychotherapy terms, we need to meet the client right where the client is.

This is even more true for school counselors who, in too many cases, are the only therapeutic help present in the life of a given traumatized child. There is a temptation to encourage children to talk about their dark secrets but, in many situations, counselors don't have the time to follow up or to allow the child to sit with the story and make sense of it. Exposing shame and bringing it to the surface is not always helpful and is sometimes damaging. As a result, some children get flooded with powerful thoughts, memories, and emotions, which can leave them increasingly anxious and feeling out of control. It is a clinical judgment as to when to encourage a child to disclose, but it is one fraught with risk if the child becomes overwhelmed. A focus on coping, self-calming, and problem-solving skills is usually a safer, more effective bet, even if it is a less dramatic and stimulating form of interaction. Many teachers and principals complain about children who are unprepared emotionally and behaviorally to return to the academic and social demands of school after counseling sessions. It is a hard balance for counselors to achieve, creating a safe space for children to talk openly but also needing to limit their disclosures so they do not become overwhelmed and dysregulated when they leave.

In addition, Hyde (2019), a philosopher and writer, raises the provocative idea that forgetting can *promote* healing rather than reflect an implicitly damaging form of denial. It depends on a host of variables, but mainly it comes down to what any specific child needs. Excavating every negative and traumatizing event the child experiences is not always helpful, although there are practitioners who believe wholeheartedly in such a process. Hyde, essentially, distinguishes between good forgetting and bad forgetting. This is something for all of us to consider as we ask children to describe their lives, their story of trauma, their fears, and their hopes for the future. The point is that we do not need to flood a child; we should observe what happens as the child puts words to various experiences. This should help guide us through the challenging labyrinth as we try to support the child in living with less shame.

The purpose of the Basic Pyramid is to develop a system around a child, a safety net, so that we do not let that child fall headlong into a state of shame. This includes identifying all the forms of help a child needs. Having access to a strong system of care outside of school—a therapist, a prescriber, a larger community of support, among others—will complement school and family support. Understanding how the brain works and developing (as well as *rehearsing*) strategies to manage feelings of being overwhelmed or, as one child put it, "swallowed up," can be a lifesaver for some children.

In ideal circumstances, therapists will share the language and strategies developed in therapy so that school staff and caregivers can develop a plan for how to cue children to use their coping skills when they are unable to access them on their own. If there is no outside therapy, the task of providing psychoeducation and helping to develop workable coping strategies falls to school counselors, a formidable challenge given their high caseloads. But it can be done.

Clearly, shame is more widespread than solely in cases of trauma. Given the unique and sometimes extreme impact it has for children with PTSD, however, finding ways to address it is essential. This will be discussed in detail in chapter 6.

CHAPTER FIVE

Shame and Lying

Even less than the connection between trauma and shame, very little has been written about shame and how it relates to the specifics of *lying*. Children's untruths, of course, do not necessarily reflect shame; there are numerous reasons for this behavior, including the obvious rationale of trying to get what one wants. Lying can also serve as an attempt to avoid responsibility, establish control, or bring harm to someone else. More specifically, Ford, King, and Hollender (1988) describe five "varieties" of lies: (1) manipulative (associated with antisocial or sociopathic people); (2) melodramatic (to be the center of attention); (3) grandiose (to win "constant approval"); (4) evasive (to avoid blame or responsibility); and (5) guilty (to avoid disapproval).

Children with trauma and shame, just like any other children, can lie for all of the reasons above. Whatever the underlying reason, lying tends to evoke a strongly negative reaction, especially when children do it. However, as many have reported, they receive muddled and inconsistent messages about whether it is entirely wrong, sometimes wrong, or, frankly, acceptable. As a result, our communications to them are complex—and confusing.

Note these contrasting quotes: There is a "real cost of even minor instances of cheating. . . . We need to be more vigilant in our efforts to curb even small infractions" (Dan Ariely); "When it comes to foreign policy, success excuses lying" (John Mearsheimer); and "Once when I was younger; in the bloom of youth; I was given an honest answer, when a lie would do" (Tracy Chapman). Whether the story has to do with students in the classroom, international affairs, or a musician's sad reflections on her relationship, these statements could not be more contradictory. It's hard for children to make sense of them since, especially during adolescence, they observe us more to see what we do than to adhere to what we tell them. According to much of the research on the subject, we lie a whole lot more than we acknowledge or perhaps even realize.

On top of this, there is the voicing of white lies, sometimes seen as the "right" thing to do but at other times called a punishable act. It is small surprise that children are baffled by our mixed messages and our insistence on their telling the truth; I have had children express exactly this. In our social and political climate, I genuinely do not know how they can begin to make sense of competing claims regarding "fake news" and malleable facts—or what these mean in terms of our expectations of them and how they should navigate their social worlds.

To complicate these ideas: If shame underlies a traumatized child's lying, such as the boy with a history of rejection and abandonment who tells false stories to try to make himself look better in the eyes of peers, the inconsistent messages about whether or not lying matters will only affirm his perception of an unsafe, chaotic world with few rules. From this perspective, a successful lie is a counterfeit victory. Increased anxiety, a lack of trust, the sense that there are few predictable rules—in short, the lack of a sturdy organizing structure to hold us—are implications. And whichever moral message we convey, it is this very behavior that lands so many children in trouble in school, at home, and, at times, with the courts. While, as noted, there are many different motives for lying, I will focus on a few aspects most closely related to shame as an emotional subset of trauma.

Over time, I have observed three primary trends. Here is one: Ekman writes, "Bald-faced lies betray and corrode closeness" (1987, p. 6). For some traumatized children with shame, that is exactly the point. It puts a hard stop to any possible intimacy, even when that same child may be yearning for deeper connections. Harris (2013, p. 41) describes lying in this way: "To lie is to a recoil from relationship." His work addresses lying as a philosophical concern rather than a clinical one, but the two overlap in meaningful ways. Lying allows a child to keep people at a safe distance, although what that child perceives as "safe" may change regularly. I know children who could be described as reflexive liars—they will lie about virtually anything—which one child told me was his way of keeping others "far away from what I really think." But the lying took on a life of its own when it became virtually automatic; this boy surprised himself at times over what came out of his mouth. In an honest moment he confided, "I'll lie about what day it is if someone asks me. I'm not even sure why." Children who display this pattern are referred to as "compulsive liars." Another child, Amanda, explained that lying allowed her to feel less threatened and more powerful in her interactions; she makes conscious choices about when to tell the truth.

Harris also notes an intriguing finding, that liars tend to *deprecate* those they lie to, which I understand to mean that, like Amanda, it lets them feel more in control of any exchange. Bok (1999) takes it a step further, referring to lying as "coercive." While this may help a traumatized child in the short-term to manage anxiety and self-esteem, it risks dehumanizing the other person. Thus, Harris's observation about lying and how it represents a kind of holding oneself away from relationships is fitting—and concerning. Coping comes in many forms, some of them useful and others less so, but this method—lying to maintain one's inner balance—comes at huge cost. Artificial relationships, mistrust on the part of others, and negative consequences for the behavior all emerge as a result. Dehumanizing other people can lead to what looks like a lack of caring at best and antisocial behavior at worst. Clearly, we need to help these children explore better avenues for taking care of themselves by developing some degree of self-compassion and maintaining safe and, at the same time, authentic relationships. As adults, we need to model the same.

A second trend, rooted in the disorganized thinking and often chaotic lives of many children with trauma, is based on a child's diminished level of social awareness. Mentalizing, theory of mind, perspective taking: these are all terms for one's capacity to recognize how others think, feel, or absorb the impact of one's actions. Whether, as we usually see in autism spectrum disorders, a child has an innate neurological challenge making sense of someone else's inner world of thoughts and emotions—and ultimately that other person's words and behaviors—or a similar challenge based on trauma, improving this skill set is critical if one is to get along successfully with others. Much of education's push for integrating SEL into classrooms and throughout schools highlights these very abilities. Children's social worlds and networks are complex. Their succeeding in comprehending what is going on around them is an essential starting point; otherwise they will be left continually trying to figure things out. This is a stressful and demoralizing process, as more than one child has told me.

As a result, traumatized children commonly struggle with how to accurately read the cues and intentions of others. This is part of an overall struggle with executive functioning and social-emotional skills. In addition, they may lack confidence in their read of others' cues, which makes sense in situations in which they have been misled by those they trusted, but it means they are prone to seeing threat or lack of caring where it may not exist. As a result, their lying, in the attempt to connect with others or foster a sense of self-protection, can sink them even more deeply into mistrust and loneliness. Therefore, they may keep other people at a distance even when they desperately seek the opposite.

Bronson and Merryman (2009) argue that some forms of lying represent a kind of advanced social skill. While they do not treat such behavior as morally justified, they report that popular, socially savvy children are the ones who lie the *most*. These children, then, are good at lying. They interpret others' cues effectively and have mastered the art form. This differs, however, from many children with trauma, whose lying represents a different tone and meaning. Two examples will clarify this distinction.

Tim, a savvy 6th grader who has somehow managed to stay out of trouble while lying consistently and skillfully to get what he wants from his peers and, often, his teachers, is remarkable both in his capacity to organize his untruths and his comfort level in using them. He sees nothing wrong in this, even though he is a nice enough kid otherwise and is not particularly mean or angry. In fact, he is well liked by other students in school. In this sense, he is a perfect example of Bronson and Merryman's description as well as Ford et al.'s reference to both "evasive" and "manipulative" liars. He explained that he views lying as something that "everyone does" and is to some degree proud that he mastered it so effectively. His joking comment was, "All people want to be the best at something, and this might be mine." At least, I hoped he was joking. We met only because he had gotten into a rare fight with another student and was required to see a consulting clinician—me—at his rural school. Tim's school counselor reports a family history of deception, with one parent having apparently lied extensively about an earlier substance abuse problem and the other about a previous, intermittent extramarital affair. For Tim, lying is something one does simply to get what one wants. To be clear, he does not present as a child with trauma. While his mother and father have their own challenging histories, there is no reported history of specific traumatizing events. He is deeply connected to his parents, and he shares in his own terms that he feels seen and cared for by both, not to mention two sets of doting grandparents.

To Tim, socially popular and a frequent flyer in the realm of lying, his ability to lie is a measure of success. It often achieves for him exactly what he wants. In clinical terms, he displays virtually no symptoms of PTSD. One might consider him "disordered" in some *DSM*-related way, but, as noted, Bronson and Merryman discuss research revealing that it is the *most* socially astute children who lie the most, almost directly in contrast with what had been predicted earlier. Without intervention, Tim is likely to remain a skilled liar. It would be intriguing to know which profession he ends up in later in life.

By comparison, 14-year-old Eric is disorganized and sometimes erratic. Living in yet another foster home—his third—he had already frustrated his very experienced foster mother within a couple of weeks of his arrival. She noted that his lies had a kind of "desperate" quality. After getting caught stealing $20 from a teacher's wallet, he wailed and denied any involvement. This was in spite of the fact that the money was found in his coat pocket. Eric ultimately confessed to the act, but it turned out that he was put up to it by two other boys in his class. Listening to his explanation, however, was a bewildering journey into his stream-of-consciousness fantasy world and deep pit of fear. There was no cohesion to his story—no beginning, middle, and end—nor was it a particularly compelling account. It was plain, if not blatantly obvious, that he had lied. It dawned on me that while Eric knew at some level that he was not telling the truth, he had constructed a story that protected him and temporarily engulfed him in the belief that he had not really done anything wrong. (Ariely's research from 2012 strongly supports the notion of self-deception as a powerful force in justifying one's lies.) The story itself was wildly inconsistent.

Once the truth was out, he was remorseful, frightened, teary, and clearly flooded with shame. He never did acknowledge that the other boys had coerced him, even though this was the reality. That information came from another child, and the two boys later admitted to it. Fitting in and having others include him surpassed everything else; the other boys were manipulating him, but Eric appeared not to recognize or acknowledge this at all. Anxious, socially immature, unable to accurately comprehend social nuances, he was an easy target. Compared to Bronson and Merryman's artful liars, Eric was the opposite.

Eric was diagnosed with PTSD at an early age along with a host of other psychiatric and developmental issues, including generalized anxiety, ADHD, and specific learning disabilities. He also had sleep difficulties. As noted, his lying was intended less in order to manipulate and more to maneuver desperately to fit in and feel part of his new school. There was a quality to his narrative that sounded like an attempt to reduce his shame and grief; this was a boy who had moved around and experienced a lot of hurt and rejection. While it does not justify stealing and lying, it was clear that his goal was to feel better—worthwhile, an integral part of things, someone who belongs—rather than to necessarily put one over on others. His remorse was real and not solely because he had been "caught." Based on Ford et al.'s categories, Eric's lies were primarily "grandiose." Being the center of attention— or, more accurately in his case, accepted by others—was something he craved, even if he had to generate false stories or engage in stealing.

It took patience on the part of the adults around him, but when Eric finally pieced together the true story for them, he bared a heartbreaking sense of humiliation. His typical pattern was to become hostile and even aggressive to get people to step back away from him. If he felt attacked, he activated his protective self and attacked others first. Exposing the lie immediately and in a confrontational, shame-inducing way had not—had never—worked with Eric. Instead, his foster mother and school principal, putting aside their own disappointment and anger, simply asked Eric about his experience of the new school and how he thought his teacher felt about the missing money. His foster mother described the look on his face as "crestfallen." Eric, in spite of the river of emotions, struck me as relieved in the telling.

On the surface, both Tim and Eric lied. But the basis for the lying was markedly dissimilar. Often, however, the consequences for getting caught are the same nonetheless, especially in school settings with a "zero tolerance" policy. To be effective, even identical presenting behaviors need to be treated in thoughtful, distinct ways, with some attempt to make sense of the meaning of the behavior (Levine, 2007). We seem to grasp this idea intuitively when it involves internalizing behaviors like anxiety or depression, but I find it much less common around the disruptive behavioral disorders such as oppositional defiant disorder (ODD) and conduct disorder (CD). Lying is a hallmark of both ODD and CD as well as of childhood trauma.

The third pattern I have observed is that of children who lie to feel in control. For some children with shame and trauma, especially those with histories of abuse, control can be a vessel hard to fill; they are continually seeking to do so. As noted, some of these children lie to maintain a sense of distance and safety in their interactions because, that way, they do not need to reveal themselves or make themselves vulnerable. Others, such as those with severe attachment issues (as in the diagnosis of reactive attachment disorder, or RAD), will lie to control *others*, which falls under the guise of manipulative lying. In this instance, the lying is more about their trauma than an internalized sense of shame, which differentiates the two to some extent. Teachers, counselors, caregivers, almost everyone can be baffled by these children and their incessant need to take control of situations, whether it is through lying or some other form of coercion. These children are often disliked for their calculating style. But it reflects their trauma. If their needs are not met during their early years, they have to get what they want and need through other means. This does not imply—at all—that they should not be held accountable for their actions. Again, we will discuss restitution in the next chapter.

I spoke with an experienced teacher, a caring, patient woman recognized in her large urban school known for making strong connections with her students. She was, in the exact word she used, "awed" by the controlling behavior of one of her students, a 5th grader we'll call Tomas. This boy had arrived a year earlier with an existing diagnosis of reactive attachment disorder, which apparently was given him during his preschool years. He was adopted from another country before he turned 11 months. (It is widely assumed that only adopted children and those in foster care can be diagnosed with RAD, but any child who has experienced early abandonment and disrupted attachment can develop it.) Tomas would lie to take advantage of almost any situation or even to orchestrate tensions among other students. At times, according to his teacher, he would "create" situations simply to then exert control over them. She described him as a kind of brilliant puppeteer in his ability to set the stage. Unlike Eric and other children who are disorganized and slower to pick up on social cues, Tomas quickly and accurately assessed almost every situation. This is an antisocial and more extreme version of lying to gain control, but it is not a unique story.

My argument is not that children with trauma necessarily lie more than other children, although that is certainly possible, if not likely. No data reliably speak to this question. Some traumatized children will lie for the same reasons as any other child, whether it is to get their own way, to boost themselves in the eyes of others, or to avoid getting into trouble. In addition, they may lie to protect the privacy of their families or to hide the stories of their abuse. Some have other serious diagnoses that lead to antisocial behavior. I have heard countless stories like Eric's in which a child with trauma wants to feel seen, appreciated, and less devalued both by peers and adults. There is typically immense pain lurking behind those lies, made worse by the reality that these children's false stories are ineffective at getting them what they want.

For many, there is a frantic need to protect their internalized sense of self-worth and significance. I have listened to elaborate, highly detailed—and made-up—stories of riches and achievements that, at times, seem critical to a child's well-being rather than embedded in a conscious attempt to manipulate others. These are a combination of Ford's "melodramatic" and "grandiose" lies. There is nothing to gain other than a temporary boost in self-esteem, but it is one built on a house of cards.

Typically, I ask children about their stories rather than attack their veracity head-on. It is tempting at times to name it, to let children know that their stories do not add up or are not even in the realm of possibility, but I hold back early on and simply express curiosity. With younger children—and sometimes this includes children up through adolescence, depending on their developmental level—I ask if the story is "truth" or "wish." I have been surprised at how many will share that, in reality, it is a fantasy, something they know they want or need, rather than something to be taken at face value. This only works when I ask in a nonconfrontational way.

By adopting this strategy, you may be accused of being "too easy" on a child who is lying to you. From a trauma-informed perspective, it is about getting to the heart of the matter and thinking carefully about variables, such as shame and the best timing for any specific conversation. You can walk around a wall of resistance more easily than bang your way through it. I have tried the latter and have the clinical bruises to show for it.

I have learned that slamming against that proverbial wall of resistance is not successful. The resistance is there for a reason, one that protects children and may have served them well as a survival strategy during their traumatic experiences. As one boy pointedly told me, "I don't give in. Ever." This included questioning his version of truth once he had dug in. Attacking their lies only entrenches children in their stories and creates fear and hostility—and, ironically, mistrust. This sometimes works in the short run—a child admits having made up the story—but it does nothing to help children figure out a better way to engage with others or reduce the chaos that ties their internal worlds together. Addressing their sadness, shame, anxiety, and, most of all, their perceived lack of safety and belonging goes much further. I know some teachers and parents who will argue that this approach serves to "enable" children, but I disagree: there are different ways to call out unwanted behavior, all of which should be based on the unique characteristics and development of any child.

In summary, shame and lying are commonly but not exclusively linked. Lying serves many purposes, but it often works as an attempt to protect traumatized children from overwhelming and painful feelings. The question, of course, is what to do when we recognize that this kind of attempt at self-protection is unfolding.

CHAPTER SIX

Making It Up to Others: Restitutional Practices

As in Eric's story, one way to combat shame, and to create opportunities for recognizing the impact of one's behavior on someone else, is to use restitution. In simple terms, this is about making it up to others when we have said or done something that hurts them in some way, which includes having lied. While there are different models and names for restitution—restorative justice and reparative justice are two of the principal ones—the term *restorative practices* is most often used to refer to the overarching concept (Wachtel, 2016). Whatever terms are used, they boil down to some shared, fundamental ideas. Primary among them is to apologize, recognize how one's words and behavior affect someone else, and accept responsibility.

While this sounds like the kind of ideal we hold for any child, it is more challenging, in some situations, for children with trauma. If your history is that "owning up" leads to violent outcomes, you quickly learn to deny at all cost. I have seen children caught in the act—one boy was *literally* holding stolen items in his hands—who swear they are not responsible. This sort of primitive denial, while it can represent other clinical issues, is not uncommon in children who have been seriously harmed for what they did and admitted to. Denial in this context becomes a survival tool, but it is one gone awry when a child needs to take legitimate responsibility in other, nonthreatening situations.

To describe their work, Fronius, Persson, Guckenburg, Hurley, and Petrosino (2019, p. 1) use the term "restorative justice," which they define as "a broad term that encompasses a growing social movement to institutionalize non-punitive, relationship-centered approaches for avoiding and addressing harm . . . and collaboratively solving problems." The authors go on to say that, in the realm of schools, the intent is to move away from "traditional discipline" and what they call "exclusionary disciplinary actions such as suspension or expulsions." This is whether one adopts formal practices such as "community circles" or more informal methods.

Whatever we call it, restitution has many benefits. For one thing, it can salvage peer relationships that might otherwise close off completely. We all want to be treated fairly and with respect. Restitution, especially when carried out in a meaningful way, raises the potential for the other person to be willing to resume the relationship. As one girl told me who had been hurt by another child's false statements—the latter was diagnosed with PTSD based on a history of abandonment when, at age six, her mother left her with an aunt and then never returned—it is hard to "turn the other cheek when someone has lied to your face and tried to embarrass you." After a little while, though, and after a heartfelt act of restitution (a public acknowledgment of responsibility, which took many rounds of rehearsal and a lot of deep breaths), they moved on as friends.

As we all know, the world of social media has only amplified the opportunities to lie about others or make disparaging comments that one might think twice about saying in person. The speed at which these comments spread is remarkable; there is no taking them back, whether they are intentionally hurtful or the result of an impulsive act. The need for restitution is even greater as a result. Otherwise, a lingering bitterness and anger can contaminate even the strongest relationships.

Another benefit, a critical one for a child's own sense of well-being, is that performing an act of restitution, whether as simple as cleaning up after destroying something or as complex as penning an honest, reflective apology note, allows the child to be *finished* with an issue. I cannot overstate the importance of this point. Traumatized children often cannot let go of poor choices they have made; they do not know how to be done with something. I have listened to whole litanies of the wrongs children have committed, and in some cases, they can ruminate almost endlessly about what they did, when they did it, and so forth. They are weighted down with what seems like a thousand bricks on their shoulders. The chance to make it up, to do something meaningful for that other person, can alleviate some of this heavy load. As a result, there may be less ongoing self-criticism, hurt, and anger.

Obviously, this does not mean that every child with trauma wants—or is even willing—to engage in such a process, but if nothing else, it creates an opening. This is entirely different from being sent to a principal's office for detention, suspension, or some other consequence that affects no one other than that specific child. It leaves the child with a lot to carry inside. Self-blame and, more severely, a crushing self-hatred can linger. These negative feelings are only exacerbated by the loss of important friendships when there is no meaningful opportunity to make it up to others and move on.

The push to improve SEL in schools is often framed as the rationale for using restitutional interventions. While a positive development, this is only part of the story, at least for children with trauma. The opportunity for children to ease their shame by restoring a broken relationship, to get back on an even keel with someone else, is one of the healthiest acts they can engage in. When successful, it reduces loss and additional rejection. And it builds on other SEL skills that may need to emerge or develop further, including recognition of others' needs and increased self-awareness.

It helps to give children the chance to contribute to deciding what their restitution should look like. It increases the likelihood that they will actively partake in the process. Children are on a continuum for their willingness/ability to accept the idea of taking this step or to participate at all. At the most extreme level, there are those who need to be pushed to provide restitution. While some may internalize nothing other than that they are able to avoid punitive consequences, it nonetheless builds in, intellectually if not emotionally, this idea: If I mistreat someone, I have to make it up directly to that person. We cannot teach any child to *feel* it internally, but we can at least supply the relevant opportunities and expectations. Maybe one way to think of this is that we are attempting to nudge the developmental process along, where children move to a higher level of ethics in which they apologize because they care about having hurt someone else rather than because they "have to."

Another reason I prefer children to weigh in on their form of restitution, a crucial one, is that we often discover what they are able—and unable—to tolerate. For example, many people with intense shame (whether related to trauma or not) are triggered by eye contact, meaning a face-to-face apology is *not* a good option. I have interviewed adults who could speak openly about this idea either as a historical or current one; many of them recount that looking directly into someone's eyes—or the other person looking straight into theirs—is like walking barefoot on hot coals. One man, now in his early 40s and a survivor of terrible trauma, met with me to talk about his troubled adolescent son. Reporting on his own history, he said that his brain "literally stopped working" when he was upset and someone looked at him too intently; he experienced it as a direct, almost primitive threat. He compared it to finding oneself among a pack of wolves and focusing only on raw survival. Even now, with the benefit of a wider view of the world and more than 40 years of life experience, he still needs to avoid eye contact when he perceives that he is getting agitated. For him, this is a coping strategy that allows him to function at work and in different social environments.

Interestingly, I find that a small percentage of young children with trauma are mistakenly categorized as having autism for this very reason; they lack eye contact during stressful or difficult interactions, which includes their face-to-face interviews with physicians, psychologists, and other mental health professionals from whom they receive a formal diagnosis. And they may erupt if eye contact is forced. What it boils down to is this: A child should perform restitution but in ways that will be successful for that child and that will also have meaning for the other, offended child. Despite our wish for this to happen, a direct, face-to-face apology is not always necessary and can be violently counterproductive.

In my experience, the restorative circles employed in a number of schools are earning mixed reviews. Many teachers and administrators share that while they appreciate the concept, the actuality of following through is challenging and inconsistent. For some children with trauma, a restorative circle can be overstimulating and threatening; again, it depends on the child. Having a one-size-fits-all approach will not work.

Overall, a study out of the Rand Corporation (Augustine et al., 2018) found "strong evidence" that a school's use of restitution has a positive effect on "teaching and learning conditions." Nonetheless, in some circles, restitution is viewed as too *soft* an approach. (This is ironic, since it is in some of the country's most challenging school districts—Oakland and Los Angeles, for example—that restorative methods previously took hold.) One teacher angrily, and anonymously, since this was said in a feedback evaluation after I gave a presentation, told me that without swift consequences, children think they have a "right" to act out and that they need to be held "accountable" for their behaviors.

I agree completely on the second point, but my belief is that this teacher misunderstood the how and why of restitution (and what accountability really means). If one believes in the possibility and the concept of a child having a skills deficit rather than displaying purposely willful behavior, such an intervention makes sense. Incentive-based behavior plans and punishment approaches, which I view as behavioral in nature, have been with us for a long time, with a mixed, if not poor, track record of success (Virues-Ortega, 2006; Kohn, 1993). This is aside from the ethical concerns that go with using them. Restitution, in comparison, is a relational approach, and for many children with trauma and related shame, it is an effective way to improve both their social-emotional skills (the awareness of others' needs) and their ability to engage in less self-blame. (Engel, 2013, argues that anything that improves self-compassion can serve as an antidote to shame.) As a result, it offers the potential to preserve their most important relationships. And it holds open the possibility for significant growth.

Restitution takes many forms and requires creativity. What one child can endure may be different from what the other child needs as an apology. The process involves reflection and teamwork, practices that can be in short supply in schools when there are dozens of issues to be dealt with all at once. I find restitutional opportunities—or what the Responsive Classroom approach calls an "apology of action"—simpler on the elementary level. For example, many teachers have classroom jobs that rotate throughout the week or month. One option is to allow the offended child the choice to swap jobs or even give an assigned job away to the other child. Or, if there is a line leader position, it can be switched. These are not time-consuming, but they can serve as concrete, meaningful, and effective strategies.

For middle- and high-school students who act in hurtful ways toward others, notes of apology are a good starting point, and I have found them to be most effective when the offended students first describe in writing the impact of that hurtful behavior. Some of the latter group are willing to open themselves up for this; others are not. I always recommend offering the choice, since any perceived power differential needs to be recognized and honored. The last thing we want to do is revictimize a child. Teachers, too, will sometimes describe the impact of a student's behavior in their classrooms in expectation of an apology; in the same way, some teachers are inclined to specifically describe the impact while others will not.

Providing feedback to the offending student about how sincerely the note comes across is also important. Some school counselors will offer such feedback, although I have also seen administrators who will do this. It is best when it is oriented as problem-solving feedback rather than positioned as a "You'd better do this or else." Avoiding power struggles whenever we can is helpful.

I am often asked what should happen if a child refuses to do restitution. I never force the issue in the moment; that would only set off another fight, flight, or freeze response. Typically, it is more effective to plan with the child when and how it will take place, even if it is later that day. If a child continually rejects the idea—something I rarely see—and was adequately prepared ahead of time (and agreed to the restitutional strategies built into the child's support plan), it may be time to use a consequence. In most situations, if it reaches this point, it usually takes just once and then the child will move to using restitution. Sometimes it makes sense to actively support the child in doing restitution, especially if it is a first time and an unfamiliar practice.

One rural, regional high school takes a creative approach to making different restitutional opportunities available to its students. One of those options lies in the simple act of where students park their cars. Parking is a highly sought-after perk, especially in my frigid weather zone, and the parking lot stretches a long way from the building. Giving up one's assigned space is not to be taken lightly, but there have been a number of instances in which this was used as a form of restitution. Some students offered it as a way to "make it up" to others and it became, in a positive way, part of the school culture.

The broader point is that restitution, however it is implemented, is helpful on multiple levels. It allows children with trauma whose actions have been harmful to others to make amends in a meaningful way and, hopefully, to move on without, as one student described it, "a lifetime of self-loathing." When conducted with sincerity, it can leave less shame and regret in its wake. It has the potential to salvage important relationships. The process, then, very much holds children accountable for their behavior, just not in the traditional sense of the word.

Finally, restitution should be built into any individualized Pyramid as an expected aspect of the plan. This removes the pressure of requesting it when things are escalated. Children know from the start that it is an integral piece and should understand that, at the end, both the one who hurts and the one who is hurt will be better off for taking such a step. If predictability is key for virtually all traumatized children, knowing about restitution and agreeing on the form it will take usually helps the process along.

CHAPTER SEVEN

Co-Occurring Diagnoses and Children's Meaning Making

The diagnosis of PTSD rarely shows up in isolation. Among children, you commonly see other psychiatric labels, especially in the category of anxiety disorders: generalized anxiety disorder (GAD), panic disorder, social anxiety disorder, separation anxiety, and various phobias. ADHD is frequent if not almost a constant. We also see depression in its many forms; mood regulation disorders, such as bipolar disorder and disruptive mood dysregulation disorder (DMDD); and occasional outbursts with the formal title of intermittent explosive disorder. In addition, there are the disruptive behavioral disorders such as conduct disorder and ODD. Interestingly, self-harm, referred to as nonsuicidal self-injury (NSSI) if there is no intent to end one's life, was not added to the *DSM* until the most recent edition, in 2013. Then there are neurodevelopmental issues such as autism spectrum disorders (ASD) and Tourette's syndrome (TS), not to mention the entire range of addictions and specific learning disabilities. In other words, there's a massive if not dizzying number of diagnostic names and labels. It is often these other diagnoses that, at least initially, lead people, children and adults alike, to seek help in therapy.

When I know that a child has experienced trauma to the extent that the symptoms qualify for a diagnosis of PTSD, I want to understand as fully as possible how it impacts that child. Intrusive or disorganized thoughts? Nightmares? Avoidance? Lying? An inability to trust others or form relationships? All of the elements discussed earlier are on the table for exploration.

At the same time, I want to know how those other diagnoses enter the picture. We need to know more than that the child has a history of trauma. Just as I rarely encounter children in practice who solely have ADHD, it is equally common to find co-occurring (or comorbid) mental health concerns among children with PTSD. If anxiety and depression are rampant, so is the lack of self-regulation linked to various mood and behavioral disorders. The point is that we need to see the entire picture, not just a list of diagnoses, and to make sense not only of the individual labels but also how they intersect and play off one another. This is where the biopsychosocial perspective is so relevant: We should address any child's biological contributors (such as medical issues), psychological factors, and social supports along with the impact of other environmental factors. Similarly, we should know about the child's strength areas so we can help the child build on those. It should not be all about focusing on problems and deficits. This has long been a criticism of psychotherapy—at least until Positive Psychology and its ideas for a strengths-based approach came along in 1998—that it emphasizes deficits rather than what is going well.

For some children with trauma, co-occurring disorders are the direct result of their lived experience. It is not hard to imagine why. The lack of control, the violation of trust, the encounters with violence and discrimination all can leave the child in a perpetual state of high alert, anxiety, and fear—or numb, angry, and depressed. Either way, the child may live in in a state of what is called *survival brain*. For these children, psychiatric labels do nothing more than reflect how they have come to survive in an unpredictable world.

This is not an established sequence. Children with PTSD may carry some of these other diagnoses *before* experiencing trauma. And while PTSD certainly lends itself to many of the diagnoses on that list, it is separate from having, for example, autism. Trauma can happen at any time, but so can the emergence of mental health struggles. Similarly, children are born with neurodevelopmental concerns even if the signs do not show up right away. Whether trauma comes before or after, it will exacerbate preexisting conditions, given the distress and disruption it causes.

Another co-occurring diagnosis: The question of personality disorders is often introduced in terms of children who have grown up in chaotic situations and then appear to "stir the pot" whenever things seem calm. It is almost as though they are unable to tolerate the lack of turbulence, given its familiarity. These children create turmoil and then may wonder why their teachers, parents, and peers are frustrated with them. The words *borderline personality disorder* strike fear in the hearts of many clinicians as it typically suggests a child who will be explosive and unpredictable. The word *manipulative* is often mentioned. I will not delve into the research on this topic, but there has long been debate as to whether we should diagnose children before the age of 18 with personality disorders. Whether there is a formal diagnostic label in place or not, their unstable relationships, intensity, and often impulsive and risky behaviors frame the stories people tell about them.

It is a delicate question, though. Diagnosing a child with borderline personality disorder may be based solely—and accurately—on presenting symptoms, but at the same time it is an inherently damaging label. Walk into any clinical or educational setting and say the following words: "The child's diagnosed as borderline." The reaction is almost universally negative. I am not in the least negating the challenges these children pose, but for many, behaviors and traits are consistent with what they know and have experienced directly. In clinical terms, this is referred to as *reenactment*, the negative behaviors that reflect a child's trauma history manifesting over and over again. Freud described the process as a *repetition compulsion*, a neurotic, ongoing—and fruitless—attempt to re-create situations to try to master them. It is a hallmark of trauma, an unfortunate one, because it can keep children stuck in a negative cycle that reinforces the belief that they are unable to get along with others or, worse, that they are unloved and unlovable. At the same time, these signs are also a significant rationale for diagnosing borderline personality disorder. Ultimately, whether a clinician applies this label to a child with PTSD may be as much a philosophical and ethical decision as it is a clinical one.

Sometimes, the *lack* of a relevant trauma diagnosis contributes to identifying and emphasizing different diagnoses in its place. For example, I met a child labeled with *alexithymia*—the inability to identify and articulate how one feels, essentially the opposite of high emotional intelligence—because he was withdrawn and usually silent. (There was also a question at one time about selective mutism, except that he said little in literally *every* setting.) As it turns out, he chose not to reveal that he had been sexually exploited nor to reflect aloud on how he was feeling or doing. His feelings of shame, when his words first emerged out of that extremely hard shell he wore around him, were profoundly entrenched. The traits of alexithymia, a condition relatively common among children with autism as well as those with various other psychiatric disorders, framed the child as incapable of knowing his emotions rather than as someone lacking trust and actively making a choice he thought might protect him. There is no substitute for getting at the full picture, or as much of it as we are able to uncover.

Whether there is a single diagnosis or multiple ones, it is helpful for children, depending on their chronological and developmental ages, to have access to this information. *How* it is presented is a key variable. If mention of PTSD is expressed in deficit language, virtually any child will recoil. It is the same with any other diagnosis. If instead it is grounded in a discussion of what is hard for them—amid observations of what they are good at—there is a much greater chance that children will want to make sense of the information and accept help. This may sound obvious, but it is not: many children either have no idea of the diagnoses they carry or have internalized them as something critically wrong and bad about them. How children know and understand is important; it is not just a simple matter of how much information we have in hand.

Meaning making. In trauma, there is also some disruption to how a child constructs meaning out of personal experiences. Emerging from humanistic branches of psychology and philosophy, those who are known as narrative, or social constructionist, theorists argue that *meaning making*, rather than the traditional psychoanalytic notions of sex and aggression, is the core human drive. Simply, we are wired to try to understand ourselves and our place in things. According to Zittoun and Brinkmann (2012, p. 1809), meaning making can be defined as "the process by which people interpret situations, events, objects, or discourses, in the light of their previous knowledge and experience . . . drawing on their history of similar situations and on available cultural resources. *It also emphasizes the fact that learning involves identities and emotions*" (emphasis added).

Kegan (1994), although he focuses more on adult meaning making, offers a critical distinction between learning new information and what he calls *transformation.* The former speaks to knowing different facts and adding to them, whether this takes the form of new content or a new set of skills. In contrast, he describes transformation as an individual radically altering "not just the way he behaves, not just the way he feels, but the way he knows— not just what he knows but the way he knows" (p. 17). In educational circles, we might describe this as similar to *metacognition*, or learning to think about how one thinks.

When it comes to traumatized children, the need to help them connect and redefine their experiences, and the emotions associated with them, is paramount so that they can create alternative ways to understand what happened, why, and where their shame comes from. One formal label given to this very human process is *cognitive reappraisal.* Narrative therapists refer to it as *restorying.* This process is, in the best instances, Kegan's notion of transformation. Whatever name we use, the purpose is to open up the possibility for children to develop a more positive identity. It does not ignore the horrors of what a child faced—if and when the child is able to go there—but it aims to integrate the child into a larger story that provides a more realistic and balanced view of what that child did or did not do. Teaching coping skills follows almost naturally when these pieces are successfully enacted. All of this is why children come to psychotherapy and, moreover, why they need a safety net of relationships that sustain them.

Pearlman (2014), also writing about meaning making in an academic vein, explains how language helps to shape our understanding of events. That is, meaning is derived from how we label and describe our own experiences. Young children who have been abused, however, may have no language at all to convey the horrors of those experiences. Or the abuse may have occurred *prior* to their development of functional language. Another potential complication is that some children will dissociate during trauma-tizing incidents and have only fragmented memories of what happened to them. Each of these scenarios shows how there may be no accessible recall that makes sense to the child or fits into a logical narrative.

Sometimes there is a complete lack of awareness that certain behaviors even constitute abuse. I once met with a child who, despite harboring huge feelings of guilt, assumed it was "normal" for young girls to have sex with their fathers because this idea is what her own father had drummed into her. Thus it is not unwillingness or "resistance"; rather, it reflects that there are no relevant words available. Pushing a child to try to articulate "what happened" or "what's wrong" can lead to an abrupt end of therapy or stop any other sig-nificant relationship in its tracks. Talk therapy, at least at the beginning of the process, is not helpful for a child who is not yet able or ready to formulate what to say.

Some children experience the expectation that they "talk about it" as not only an impossible task but even as another kind of coercion. One child angrily told me he wanted to "punch out every adult who corners me in an office and says I should talk just because they say they can be trusted." (He added a few pointed expletives to the end of this statement.) As someone naturally inclined toward drawing, this was ultimately how he shared the details of what he had endured. This is also how he made sense of his trau-matic past, by creating cartoon characters and allowing them to discover and articulate connections among events about which he had essentially stayed silent because he did not have the words to express them verbally. At one point, he told me that the characters in his drawings "taught him what really happened," a striking observation that I needed time to ponder before real-izing how significant it was.

The rich details of the characters in his pictures—and their dramatic stories—were in startling contrast to his sparse words. (I think he was delighted as well at my obvious awe of his art skills, especially because my own drawings are, to put it kindly, poor.) I could see his bitterness toward the world start to evaporate as he slowly began to construct and describe a different story about his role in events. He was fully in control of the process, how much to reveal, and when, and significantly, he could make decisions about how to understand what had happened. As he later told me, he could reserve his hatred "for the person who deserved it." This was good progress for a child whose fundamental assumption was that others would betray him and, as a result, he should necessarily "hate them first."

Attempts at new meaning making, according to narrative therapists, sup-port self-compassion and improved mental health by focusing on strengths and efforts aimed at resilience rather than the what's-wrong built into diag-nostic labels. This is not a criticism of the importance of accurate diagnostic work; however, I do have concerns about how psychiatric diagnoses are sometimes used to shape the discussion with children about their "problems" and deficits. For children with trauma, a balanced self-understanding is critical to well-being.

Knowing they are not responsible for their own abuse may sound like an obvious goal, but for many children, grasping it emotionally as well as intellectually is infinitely more of a challenge. Again, this is especially complicated when children have been told, sometimes repeatedly (this happens frequently in cases of ongoing sexual abuse), that they were the cause. In these instances, even a short conversation will often expose a powerful distortion of their thinking, emotions, and formulation of meaning. At times, you can find yourself disoriented and thinking that there are two entirely separate realities under consideration.

This complexity comes to life when you ask severely traumatized children to tell you something good about themselves. Some children have nothing to say and seem confused by the question, others squirm uncomfortably, and others might report a positive comment said about them by someone else, that is, a third-person compliment that the children do not have to own for themselves. Those who can identify their strengths may seem at times to not even be referring to themselves. Individually, they may distance themselves from "that child" who does good things, can express kindness, or has talents. Acknowledging a strength or positive attribute, especially when they are lashed to a harsh, self-blaming view, does not fit with the meaning they have created about their lives and their place within them. It causes cognitive dissonance. It may take a long time before such children can comfortably accept those strengths as their own.

These comments about meaning making underlie the discussion in the next chapter of psychotherapy with traumatized children and, later, how meaning making can be oriented to contributing toward what is known as post-traumatic growth. All of this will return us to the value in using the Basic Pyramid in thoughtful, systematic ways.

Psychotherapy for Children with Trauma

Some of the clinical approaches used in therapy settings can be adapted by school staff and caregivers as part of developing a Pyramid for any particular child. Many of them focus on helping children learn different ways to manage their overwhelming physiological responses to stress. Given the emotional (survival) brain response to incoming stories, events, and other triggers among children with trauma, some of our intervention needs to be geared to helping the body avoid its habitual five-alarm response. As one adolescent told me unhappily and with an intense look directly into my eyes (extremely unusual for him), this is easier said than done. He knows what to do but struggles over how to apply it in the moment. I have heard this same comment countless times from adults as well as children with PTSD.

This susceptibility to emotional responding seems especially true during contentious political periods. Davies (2018), a political economist, wrote a book showing how, even on the political level, we experience events—and make critical decisions—based on "gut feelings" rather than what we might consider rational thinking. If this is true for mature adults granted positions of power in our culture, imagine how this might fit for children with trauma. We are modeling not thoughtful consideration but heightened, rapid-fire emotional tirades directed at perceived threats—whether they exist or not. Many children with trauma end up doing exactly the same. They watch what we do, observe how we perform under pressure, and try to interpret the different ways we cope.

Another economist, Kahneman (2011) wrote a Nobel Prize-winning book distinguishing between what he calls System 1 and System 2 thinking. In short, the latter is the slow, careful analysis needed to make a reasoned decision. In contrast, System 1 thinking is quick, instinctive, and reliant on pattern recognition. We scan a situation, link it to what we know from prior experience, good or bad, and decide/act accordingly. While this saves time in reaching a conclusion, it also means that we often depend too strongly on our intuitions, past experiences, and snap judgments, which is especially problematic if we consistently tend to perceive hostility and threat. Or, for some children, it is the opposite: they lack the necessary awareness of risk when it is warranted, sometimes due to a history of powerlessness. Some find themselves in dangerous situations with little real sense of how they ended up there. System 1 thinking may be faster, but it offers limited opportunity to effectively assess all of the possible options in more complex situations. Clearly, emotional responding reflects this version.

It may seem surprising that the two researchers I referenced so far are economists rather than behavioral health specialists. However, understanding how we process information and then react is critical to numerous fields of study. This, of course, includes mental health, where we continue to work on finding ways to counter the intense responses we see in many children with trauma. Both Davies and Kahneman point to the need to offset our powerful first reactions and think through how we want to proceed, whether our decision-making has to do with politics, medicine, finances, or any other area of our lives. This is especially important for children with trauma, who frequently reside in a state of hyperarousal and end up exacerbating the problems they are trying to solve. That is, their usual coping skills, their careful watching and readiness to respond to any perception of threat, lead to greater conflict with others and often within themselves.

I think of the outcome of good therapy for children with PTSD as similar to defragging a computer. For those of you unfamiliar with this computer term, it is a way to clean up your computer's hard drive. The procedure takes pieces of information dispersed throughout the hard drive and, in essence, lines them up in a logical sequence. It organizes these fragmented chunks and brings them together so that the hard drive—the computer's "brain"— can process more efficiently and effectively. The parallel, I hope, is clear: One of the goals of therapy is to help children take those disconnected fragments of memory and begin the sometimes grueling process of linking them into a coherent story. In short, the children create new meaning out of their past experiences but at a pace at which they can retain control.

For this to happen, though, children need to first learn how to manage those giant emotional waves that can physiologically overwhelm them. This hyperarousal, of course, is not what every child with trauma experiences, but it is a common enough occurrence that it is frequently the presenting complaint. Statements such as "I'm overwhelmed," "I have trouble thinking clearly," and "I have no idea what to do" reflect this state. Or the child is unable to talk at all. On the externalizing side, erratic behavior and observations that a child is "out of control" may result. Delving into traumatizing events without the skills to cope with powerful reactions can lead children to greater anxiety, disorganized thinking, a mass of painful emotional states, and the full array of behaviors that reflect a PTSD diagnosis.

While there are numerous models of psychotherapy, I want to highlight a few of them here because I believe they are some of the most relevant ones to helping children who struggle significantly with their emotional regulation. Each model has a strong evidence base behind it, which is also a critical factor. At the outset, I want to note that I am not suggesting that schools offer formal psychotherapy sessions; instead, it is that these models lend themselves to being translated into ongoing interventions that schools and, in some cases, caregivers can provide. They work well outside of therapy settings when carefully adapted to each different environment and can also be integrated into *how* we talk with children about using the Pyramid as a coping tool.

Cognitive behavioral therapy (CBT) is the most heavily researched model in psychotherapy (David, Cristea, and Hofmann, 2018). Its founding is credited to Aaron Beck during the 1960s. CBT aims to help people recognize how their thoughts can go awry rather than guide them to accurately understand events, other people, or themselves. In psychological language, their reality testing is impaired, which ultimately can lead to faulty decision-making.

In addition, a term we often hear is *catastrophizing*, which is when we take an average problem and turn it into an end-of-the-world crisis. This happens frequently in cases of trauma—and in anxiety and depression as well—because one's capacity to accurately gauge the size of any issue may be reduced. When you are under severe stress, even the most minor challenge may seem like an enormous problem. Similarly, the smallest setback can cause a furious reaction. These are common outcomes when someone's thinking has—in the words of one depressed young man with a long trauma history—"gone off the rails."

The approach, in short, is to help people understand their automatic thoughts and how they link to their behaviors and emotions. Rather than initially focusing on feelings, which is often overstimulating and threatening for children with trauma, the primary emphasis is on finding ways to gently challenge and then modify their thinking. As a result, the goal is to improve their reality testing.

A number of models have been developed for conducting in-school CBT, but these require a potentially lengthy commitment of time from both the child and the counselor. When the opportunity exists, it can significantly benefit traumatized children, but most counselors simply do not have enough space in their schedules—or, necessarily, sufficient training—to conduct formal therapy sessions. Instead, elements of CBT can be employed by counselors in their brief meetings with these children, looking especially at the question of *how* a dysregulated child routinely comes to particular conclusions and trying to help that child shift to Kahneman's slower paced, more reflective System 2 way of thinking. Offering that child a different way to interpret an interaction—an opportunity for the child to alter meaning making—whether it is with a teacher, caregiver, or peer, can introduce a new understanding. It takes time and practice to reach this point.

Asking a child how big a problem the child is facing is a basic CBT strategy. I use a 1-to-5 number scale; some practitioners will use colors instead What tells the child that the problem is so large? Is there any evidence to the contrary? In short, this approach teaches children to consider whether their perceptions of threat are accurate and to stop long enough to assess a situation from various angles before acting on their emotional impulse. I have seen children catch themselves; one girl, Mabel, even started laughing good-naturedly at herself and said, "There I go again, overreacting to stuff." A comment like this tells us when the process is beginning to succeed. In the past, trying to talk Mabel out of an emotional response—or an emotional argument—virtually never worked; any parent and teacher is likely to say the same about some other child. Reacting with anger to a traumatized child's emotions is almost a surefire failure, but we are human and it happens. CBT, then, prioritizes reaching a child through the thinking process rather than the child's emotions and behaviors. It teaches children that thoughts are just that—thoughts, not necessarily a complete reflection of reality—and can change. For some children, this works to diminish their immediate flare-up.

Dialectical behavior therapy, or DBT, is a modified version of CBT developed during the latter part of the 1980s by Marsha Linehan. Similar to CBT, there have been attempts to create adapted versions that can be used with children and in schools. (For the latter, see Mazza et al., 2016.) While it is a comprehensive model that follows specific rules as to how it is structured during psychotherapy, DBT rests on some fundamental principles. An integral one is helping people who self-harm and those who display signs of borderline personality disorder—again, both are common among children with severe trauma—learn ways to better manage their emotional pain. Without what these practitioners call "distress tolerance," every issue is likely to blow up into an even larger one. An essential focus in DBT is to teach self-calming and mindfulness skills to improve daily if not moment-to-moment coping.

Another offshoot of CBT is prolonged exposure therapy. The concept of exposing people to their fears and phobias was introduced in the late 1950s by the behaviorist Joseph Wolpe. He proposed doing this gradually, via a process he called systematic desensitization. Later, during the 1990s, Edna Foa created an alternative version, prolonged exposure (or PE), which also aims to help people learn how to confront their terrors rather than avoid them. She chose a less incremental method in the belief that learning to sit with one's worst fears is the most effective way to learn to manage them. This model, along with one other (cognitive processing therapy, or CPT), is the evidence-based approach adopted by the Veterans Affairs Administration to help veterans. Since avoidance is such an integral aspect of PTSD—and, according to virtually any theory of psychotherapy, avoidance only adds to anxiety and depression—Foa's work supports bringing people directly and safely into contact with their most dreaded memories and worries. The idea is that by experiencing these memories while practicing relaxation strategies they have rehearsed beforehand, people learn how to better cope with their internal reactions and stand face-to-face with their fears rather than shut down, flee, or escalate to aggression. This allows them to function better overall, with less ongoing stress and avoidance. Prolonged exposure strategies have been adapted for use with children, especially in terms of dealing with phobias but also with respect to intrusive thoughts and memories.

A specific form of CBT developed specifically to address trauma is known as trauma-focused cognitive behavior therapy, or TF-CBT. According to Cohen and Mannarino (2008, p. 158), the acronym PRACTICE summarizes the therapy's components, which the authors identify as follows: "Psychoeducation, Parenting skills, Relaxation skills, Affective modulation skills, Cognitive coping skills, Trauma narrative and cognitive processing of the traumatic event(s), In vivo mastery of trauma reminders, Conjoint child-parent sessions, and Enhancing safety." This is a 12- to 18-session module—although the number can be increased for children with complex and severe trauma—geared to assisting caregivers as well as directly helping children. Its value lies mainly in its attention to how to teach children the skills to manage strong emotions and then process events. Thus it emphasizes the critical notions of safety and ways of coping. It is an approach like this that we hope all children with severe trauma will be given the opportunity to access, with pertinent skills then shared with school staff and other caregivers.

As I said earlier, there are forms of CBT that have been introduced into schools as adapted treatment models. A specific version centered on helping children with trauma is cognitive behavior intervention for trauma in schools (CBITS). Developed in the 1990s by a team from UCLA, the RAND Corporation, and, notably, the Los Angeles Unified School District (receiving direct input from those working in schools is a significant benefit), the idea behind CBITS is to address trauma directly within the school setting. While there is research support for the standardized model—the Substance Abuse and Mental Health Services Administration (SAMHSA) identifies CBITS as an evidence-based approach—having enough clinician time to implement it is the same challenge we see in trying to offer any kind of intensive mental health intervention within schools. Rural schools, as virtually anyone who works in one knows, often lack such resource time, but this is common almost anywhere.

Nonetheless, an appealing aspect of the model is that along with individual and group sessions (and two psychoeducation sessions for parents), there is also an educational session for teachers and other staff. This last aspect is critical, just as it would be for any Tier 3 support. It is exactly the piece that is missing in many school-based clinical services. Collaborating with the people who spend the most time with a traumatized child should be the goal for any clinician, and the Pyramid is a vehicle for taking those ideas and translating them into an action plan that everyone involved with a child can use.

The risk in using such a model is that it has the potential to trigger certain children who then are unprepared to reenter their classrooms and other activities. As always, it comes down to different variables, mainly the capacity of the child to do this work and the skill of the clinician in helping the child to manage uncomfortable thoughts and emotions. If nothing else, we should not ignore the potential for leaving a child feeling disrupted and poorly equipped to step into high-demand situations such as the classroom. One child, Rebecca, compared this scenario to a "bad swimmer getting thrown into the deep end of the pool and told to stay there. You're not allowed to leave."

One of the strengths of any form of CBT is that it demystifies the process of therapy. Children understand from the outset that learning new ways of thinking—and thus discovering new ways of feeling and acting—will only come with time and practice. At the same time, it offers a sense of control because it tells children that these are achievable skills, not special talents they lack as though they were somehow born without them. In other words, as one adolescent girl openly wondered, they are not "ordained as deficient." Although Carol Dweck's notion of a "growth mindset" is a regular topic of discussion in schools, it is almost always applied to conversations about academic growth and perseverance in a learning context. It is similar in this vein as well; children can create a gentler relationship with their intrusive, angry, self-blaming, and helplessness-inducing thoughts by developing the new skills they need.

A different therapeutic model is accelerated experiential dynamic therapy (AEDP). Without delving too far into the history and practices of psychodynamic or analytic therapies, I want to mention this approach mainly because it defines itself as a theory of change model rather than a theory of psychopathology. In other words, it rests on the notion of *neuroplasticity*, the idea that our brains are intrinsically ready to expand and grow in healthy ways when we live in a safe, nurturing environment. Thus the model focuses less on our disorders and underlying flaws. First created by Fosha (2000), it has undergone many revisions throughout the years but is consistently based on the same set of core values. There is not a specific set of "techniques" that can be adapted for caregiver or educator settings, but its fundamental beliefs are relevant to how we communicate the benefits of the Pyramid and the ways in which it can help support a child's progress. It is not only a matter of what we say to any child, it is equally a matter of what we believe. This model, in short, promotes optimism and hope.

In contrast to AEDP and the various versions of CBT, other approaches are more body-and sensory-focused. Memories of trauma can be stored anywhere, not solely in one's mental memory. This critical idea was the basis for Van der Kolk's book title, *The Body Keeps the Score* (2014). He recognized that distressing incidents can be remembered and experienced as both mental suffering and physical pain. He also described the heightened risk to one's health and well-being by living with ongoing high levels of stress and hyper-arousal. Given this, Van der Kolk was one of the early advocates for treating trauma by means of the body as well as the mind.

Before exploring a few of the specific sensory approaches to intervention, it is worth noting this idea: A different way of understanding our physical selves is by expanding our awareness of our various senses. Almost anyone will identify the five primary ones: sight, sound, taste, smell, and touch. Some will cite two others: vestibular (balance) and proprioceptive (movement through space). Mahler (2016), an occupational therapist, refers to an eight sense, "interoception," which she argues is how we experience our internal body states. More specifically, she alludes to such specific variables as hunger/fullness, thirst, pain, heart and breathing rate, social touch, and even itchiness and needing to use the bathroom.

Interestingly, she reports that the term was first used in beginning of the 20th century but that it remained relatively unknown (and unstudied) until a neuroscientist, Craig, began to study it more closely during the 1990s. Perhaps, again, this reflects the evolving movement during that decade to delving more fully into how we understand our bodies and physiological states. This is in contrast to focusing exclusively on the brain in relation to our feelings and behaviors. It was almost as if we saw humans divided into two distinct rather than intersecting parts: the mind, and everything else located below the neck. While Mahler grounds her discussion of interoception in developmental concerns such as autism, it can—and should—be applied as well to children with trauma.

For example, children in a state of severe dissociation may shut down to the point where they do not recognize their internal body states. They may wet themselves, forget to eat or drink, be unaware of cold or heat, or fail to identify body pain. I once saw a severely shut-down child come through the psychiatric emergency room for assessment who had broken her ankle; no one knew about it until the following morning, when a teacher noticed that she appeared to be limping and sent her to the nurse's office. X-rays followed, and they revealed the fracture. This child, literally, had shared nothing suggesting pain located in that area. If we view these examples of restricted internal awareness as a loss of self-regulation rather than as resistant behaviors to be "shaped" or disciplined, our interventions will reflect our grasp of the mind–body connection. And they will recognize the distinct lack of safety many traumatized children experience, which contributes to keeping them blocked and dysregulated.

One example of therapy geared to our physical sense of self is called sensory psychotherapy, an approach first developed by Pat Ogden in the 1970s. In short, it helps children (and adults) learn about the connections among their physiological states, experiences, and unconscious memories. It works to integrate these fragmented sensations and memories into a more cohesive understanding. Again, it is a kind of meaning making but one that begins with focusing on bodily sensations as opposed to thoughts or feelings. Unlike cognitive and emotionally focused approaches, this is more of an outside-in way of working. Consistent with Van der Kolk's theory, it honors the idea that our bodies hold a kind of intrinsic knowledge of our experience. Using self-awareness strategies such as meditation and mindfulness—Ogden was an early proponent—her objective is to help children understand their unique mind–body connections and cope more effectively with life's ups and downs.

Another kind of sensory-based therapy is Peter Levine's model known as somatic experiencing. It was first developed in the late 1970s and has gone through various refinements since then. Just as in sensory psychotherapy and similar to other body-based interventions such as EMDR, it also recognizes that memories of trauma are held in the body as well as the mind. Levine proposes that these memories are manifested through our autonomic nervous system, part of the larger nervous system that operates primarily on an unconscious level and helps to regulate processes such as respiration and heart rate. This model of therapy helps children with trauma by attempting to determine where they are "stuck" in their fight, flight, or freeze responses; it then applies different interventions to loosen what Peter Levine refers to as "fixated physiological states" (2010). As should be clear, the model aims to help with self-regulation, resulting in better coping skills rather than the excessive if not extreme reactions associated with fight, flight, or freeze.

A less common intervention that has been shown to help children reduce the intensity of their hyperarousal is hypnosis, or self-induction. Perry and Szalavitz (2017) describe its use in one of their case studies as a child-friendly method for creating an internal sense of peace and safety. This is not necessarily an approach that can be easily adapted into the fast pace of school settings, but as children learn to use it, they may be able to apply it themselves in different situations, including schools, when they can pull themselves out to a quiet location for a few moments. On the research side, an international study found that hypnosis is successful in reducing the symptoms of PTSD

(Rotaru and Rusu, 2016). I know few practitioners who teach children this tool, but it appears to be a worthy complement to our other interventions.

In general, the integration of sophisticated CBT-oriented and body-focused interventions represents what Siegel and Bryson (2011) call a "whole brain" approach. Although theirs is a highly simplified version—while also grounded in an understanding of existing brain research—they identify some of the important concepts related to calming a reactive, agitated child. For example, one of their tenets is to "engage not enrage," generally by using a soothing tone and a gentle touch (when it is appropriate) and focusing on helping the child to reenlist the rational "upstairs brain." These ideas, emerging out of different philosophies about children's development and the best interventions to help them, are consistent in emphasizing de-escalation and supporting the child in navigating overpowering emotions. For many children with PTSD, this is the overriding challenge.

Family therapy is an integral treatment model for supporting children as well as their caregivers. Just as it is important for teachers to have tools for helping traumatized children, it is equally essential for caregivers, whether parents, relatives, or foster parents, to have them. Educating caregivers about trauma, working on de-escalation strategies, and reestablishing positive forms of family communication are all critical. Caregivers and children can work together to create a Pyramid that fits with the specifics of each individual home setting. If there is to be a total healing environment for the most traumatized children, helping *all* involved adults will support such a process.

There are dozens of other therapeutic models and approaches designed for working with children, but these examples of CBT and body-oriented frameworks all center on a similar goal: more planful, System 2 responses and fewer extreme reactions to even the typical stresses of childhood. In addition, each model can be adapted for school staff and caregivers and incorporated into the language of the Basic Pyramid. As noted, the ideal is when an outside therapist can work intensively with traumatized children and share successful strategies with school personnel and caregivers. What gets lost at times is the idea that it is equally important for these outside providers to take into account the observations shared by people who regularly see and interact with the child. This kind of collaborative, reciprocal effort is clearly an important best-practice approach, one that appears eminently logical on the surface but is missing far too often in practice.

Adapting Therapeutic Models to Other Settings

When CBT strategies are employed in schools, the message communicated to children should be similar to what they hear in a therapist's office: A child can learn and apply new skills to cope with stresses and disappointments.

One way for schools and caregivers to help children with PTSD transfer these new skills from the therapist's office to real-life settings is to make time to delve into them and their specific fit within each different setting. This may sound obvious, but I can tell you from many years of experience that it does not happen often enough. I view the process as this: The therapist introduces skills, and children rehearse them in that safe setting, finding which ones work best and are most comfortable to use; school counselors review these skills and help children think through how to utilize them; and teachers are shown specific ways to remind their students to apply them. It is the same process for caregivers to use at home, although they often need to rely directly on the outpatient therapist for guidance, especially when there is no school counselor involved with the child.

In clinical terms, CBT is very much about improving a child's reality testing. Understanding how your thinking can lead directly to anxiety, depression, and, notably, poor decision-making is critical, even if your body is reacting strongly and, as one child framed it, "with a mind of its own." It is all about learning and rehearsing (sometimes repeatedly) strategies rather than depending on some sort of aha moment or magical intervention. Body-based interventions, on the other hand, bring awareness to blocked-off memories and emotions, reflecting the significance of the intrinsic mind–body connection and the power of the body to hold important information. I once saw a child who had unexplained leg pains; later, it was determined that she had been kicked in the shins when she was a "bad little girl" many years before.

Using a combination of CBT and body-focused approaches in schools or at home means we should ask some version of the following questions at a developmental level that fits the child. Obviously, not all of these questions can or should be asked at any one time; it is a judgment call based on the child's tolerance and willingness to engage in self-reflection. But these are the kinds of questions that signify an integration of the two different clinical approaches:

- How strongly did your fight, flight, or freeze instinct kick in?
- How big a problem do you think this situation actually was?
- What parts of your body reacted? How did you experience these sensations? Where? What do you think your body's reactions were telling you?
- What were you thinking about when you reacted? Or, conversely, were you able to think things through at all?
- What do you think the other person was thinking/feeling?
- Were you able to remember some of your calming strategies before reacting in the moment? If so, which ones? Which worked best and which the least? What did your body feel like when you tried these strategies?

- Could you adjust your own behavior when the other person first acted or responded?

- If you reacted mainly out of your emotional brain, how long did it take for you to turn off (or reduce the level of) your alarm system? What worked to help you do this? Similarly, what helped you to remember to do this?

- How did things end? How did you leave it with the other person/people? Would it help for you to apologize for anything you said or did?

- If you are confronted with this situation again tomorrow, what would help you to handle it differently (if necessary)?

- What are you thinking right now while we are reviewing all this?

- What is your anxiety level while we are talking this through? Where do you experience that anxiety? Grade it on a 1-to-5 scale, if possible.

This is not an exhaustive list, but the questions are examples of how to explore both the child's thoughts and physiological reactions. Asking about the size of the problem and the degree of anxiety models the idea of looking at things in relative terms. Issues should not be polarized as either completely unimportant or a massive concern; there is plenty of room in the middle between these two endpoints, but many children with trauma have difficulty coming to that realization. Some children need help as to how to address these questions. Others are unable to reflect on them at all.

Another theory that speaks particularly well to adapting any clinical model to school or home is called "control mastery." It is not a new approach. Begun in the 1960s by Weiss and Sampson, although their book was not published until 1986, it is still in use today even though it is not one of the more well-known psychological theories. Weiss and Sampson's perspective is that control mastery is not necessarily a specific model of intervention although it can be used in that manner. Instead, they view it as a humanistic model for understanding how people arrive at their "maladaptive beliefs"; as such, they consider it relevant to any model of therapy, including CBT. They suggest that underlying any of its specific ideas and strategies is the belief that fundamentally, we all strive toward good health and mastery of both our conscious and unconscious fears; so in some ways, it is an early example of positive psychology. That is, it has an optimistic orientation. It normalizes that we all have struggles but points to how, most of all, we aim for optimal good health. This theory, I believe, is directly applicable to so much of how we might interact even moment-to-moment with traumatized children. The parallels should be clear: We try to help children feel safe by joining them in sitting with their fears, validating them, and, at the same time, gently questioning their interpretation of events. Such a process is beneficial whether this takes place in school or at home. The similarities with CBT should be clear, although this model speaks more clearly to how, emotionally rather than cognitively, we promote children's safety.

An essential aspect of the theory lies in its founding hypothesis that only if we help children feel safe can they lift their usual psychological "defenses" and allow new meaning making to occur. (Weiss and Sampson use the term "interpretations" but they are psychoanalytically oriented thinkers and practitioners. In our context, meaning making is a more apt term.) These defenses include issues such as severe denial and blaming others for their own challenges (projection). Expecting children to quickly give up these ways of coping is unrealistic, but the giving up can and does emerge over time. In school language, it is about scaffolding, just as we assume in every child's academic path.

Formally, the model, like virtually every other clinical model, is based on the idea of doing this work in therapy. But critically for children with PTSD, it can also happen incrementally as a result of ongoing interactions with caring adults. To be clear, it is not simply a matter of being nice. Instead, it implies that our unwavering support is what counts: the clarity of our expectations, our ability to establish predictability and reasonable limits, our consistent attempts to teach skills rather than default to threats of discipline, and our understanding of context and the meaning of a child's behavior. All of these underlie a child's growing ability to see things in new and healthier ways. It is anything but a linear process—and goodness knows, we all struggle, get tired or overwhelmed, and make mistakes—but it matters. A basic premise of the model is that children will test us to see if we mean what we say. By our staying with them, avoiding shaming and abandonment, they have the opportunity and space to improve. They develop better control over their "mental content" and greater mastery of their life challenges. I have seen countless instances of this kind of progress.

To extend these ideas, I want to stress that caring and support do not mean we never get angry with a child. It happens. What is significant is how we take responsibility for it, apologize, and model how to cope with having "blown it." One boy, Jerod, later told me he trusted me *more* after I raised my voice at him—yes, this constitutes having blown it, especially given the surprising and excessive volume I used at the time—because he had been out all night and put his struggling single father into a state of panic. It had not been planned on my part. I immediately apologized, but Jerod, after looking stunned, started to laugh good-naturedly. "It's good to see that side of you, Doc," he said. As his mother, who eventually died of a drug overdose, routinely used to hit him, I think he felt relieved that my anger reached its limit in loud words—and that I did not disappear suddenly from his life. My anger, as I discovered later, also told him I genuinely cared, because he typically found clinicians to be "too nice." In other words, we can repair our human mistakes and not aim to be perfect in our roles. Many teachers and caregivers have voiced similar concerns, that they worry about having made unforgivable errors, but this is rarely the case. It is what happens *next* that determines the progression of the relationship. Whether it is about building relationships, performing in school, or playing sports, trying too hard to be perfect, to avoid making any kind of mistake, typically leads to a worse outcome.

Powerful feelings of rejection and abandonment—the "unbearable aloneness" mentioned at the outset—are common among children who have been physically, emotionally, or sexually abused. Our ability to "stay in there," to somehow avoid repeating the message that they are beyond help, is crucial. It can be exhausting work, and teachers as well as counselors may not see the fruits of their labors. I can assure you, however, that many children will talk retrospectively about adults from years earlier who, in the words of one boy, "stuck it out." Tim, an adolescent who survived some harrowing times growing up with his family, commented on a 5th-grade teacher that he credits for helping him turn the corner. Since I still occasionally consult to his old elementary school, I asked him for permission to raise his name with her. He was fine with this, but he jokingly assumed she would not have good or even decent memories of him, if she remembered him at all. When I spoke with her, her face immediately brightened. She recalled him in full, both his strengths and his struggles. She thought she had "done very little" for him, and I commonly hear this refrain from teachers who do not get to experience or witness any later progress a child demonstrates. She was delighted when I explained the current version of the little boy she remembered. And she was overjoyed—not to mention thoroughly surprised—that he still held fond memories of her.

Another example comes from an esteemed colleague of mine. Many years ago, she was a social worker for an agency in New York that provides foster care services for children. There was one 10-year-old girl with whom my colleague spent a lot of time as her caseworker. They shopped for clothes, traveled to doctor appointments, and even went to a new foster home together. Despite all her attempts to establish a connection, the child barely if ever spoke directly to her. A few years later, however, this child told a peer how wonderful a person my colleague was, saying that the other child was lucky to work with her. This woman, equal parts patient and determined, somehow managed to communicate the message that she would not reject her, no matter what.

I think of this process as laying the foundation without necessarily seeing the house built above it, but you cannot have the end result without putting in the initial work. As such, Jennings's (2019) advocacy for "compassion" for traumatized children is directly relevant here. This is challenging stuff, and it translates to not only the *what* of the Basic Pyramid but also *how* we communicate around it.

No matter which therapeutic models we adapt and use in schools, the need for teamwork and planning cannot be overstated. Again, if there is no outside therapist, it is up to a school counselor to try to creatively weave in the time to help children strategize. If nothing else, coming in from the outside, I want to know at least those three to five self-calming strategies any specific child might use. In reminder, there should be a limited number of students who need this level of intervention. It is essential for those who do and are the "heavy hitters," which is not a particularly complimentary term, but everyone who works in schools knows exactly what it signifies and can identify the children who need the most support and demand the most attention. Otherwise, everyone, including the child, is left to freelance based on what is happening in the moment. It is this very lack of structure that we would not begin to accept on an academic level or in virtually any other realm, such as playing competitive sports or learning music. For children with trauma, it is equally if not more important that the approach to helping them with their self-regulation and behavior is clearly defined.

Earlier this year, I gave a workshop to a large group of school administrators. A number of them were not particularly pleased with some—if not much—of what I had to say. No matter how much I emphasized the profoundly relational nature of helping children with trauma, their comments came back to "give us more strategies." Clearly, I was not successful enough in getting the point across that any technique, if it is to work effectively, has to be immersed in a network of meaningful, supportive relationships. We sometimes assume, from our own vantage point, that this is already in place. From a child's perspective, this may not be the case at all. Change comes from us as well as from children themselves, and often in tandem. We cannot simply fix and bend them into better shape. Watch two adults implement the same behavior plan with the same student: It may work for one and fail miserably for the other. A major variable is the presentation—the tone of voice, body language, and emotional regulation—of the adult. Strategies absolutely matter; so do the adults using them.

One practitioner of what is called polyvagal theory (Dana, 2019, p. 20, referring to Porges's work introduced in 1994) points out that our "rapid response survival system is orchestrated by our autonomic nervous system (ANS)." Without diving too far into the language of neurology, the main point is that it is the state of *both* people operating within an interactive system that creates safety—or the lack of it. How often have we seen children, or any of us for that matter, negatively affected by the subtle or overt mood of someone else? If a teacher or caregiver is highly stressed or angry, children, especially those with trauma, who are primed to observe their surroundings carefully, can quickly become upset or dysregulated.

This is not about blame. Rather, it is about self-awareness and a willingness to look as closely at ourselves as we do the behaviors of these struggling children. Siegel (2012) refers to this as "interpersonal neurobiology," the impact two individuals have on one another in reciprocal fashion. In simple terms, children do not operate in a vacuum, yet our interventions often represent exactly that perspective. Through the quality of our relationships, or what Ginwright (2018) refers to as "healing centered engagement," we are integral to their growth, the very point I could not adequately deliver in my talk to that group of educators. Whether or not we believe this or accept it as a significant aspect of what we often refer to as "behavior management," we are a critical part of the change process beyond their academic learning. Perry (2017), a child psychiatrist who works extensively with traumatized children, emphasizes this same idea.

Integrating These Approaches into the Basic Pyramid

Thinking more about these different theories and intervention models, how do we fit them, in practical terms, into the ways we use the Pyramid? What is their relevance, and how can they be adapted to children's ongoing interactions with their teachers (as well as other school staff) and caregivers?

First, the following data make clear why these questions are important. Overall, only a slim majority of children with diagnosed mental health disorders see a licensed therapist. An interesting finding is that different disorders lead to widely disparate percentages of children receiving treatment (Ghandour et al., 2019). For example, almost eight in 10 children (78.1%) ages three to 17 years old with depression receive treatment; six in 10 children (59.3%) ages three to 17 years old with anxiety (the most common diagnosis in childhood) receive treatment; and just over five in 10 children (53.5%) ages three to 17 years old with behavior disorders receive treatment. (PTSD is formally categorized as an anxiety disorder.)

Unfortunately, what we do not know from these data is how many children with these different diagnoses receive only medication, only therapy, or both. Nor is there reliable data indicating the percentage of children specifically with PTSD who are receiving therapy, but too many are not getting it. According to the Presidential Task Force on Posttraumatic Stress Disorder and Trauma in Children and Adolescents (2008), "Most children with distress related to trauma exposure and in need of help do not receive psychological treatment, and those who do receive a wide variety of treatments." I have not been able to find updated treatment data specific to PTSD since the task force issued its findings, even after reaching out to authoritative resources such as the National Child Traumatic Stress Network. Clearly, this is an area for further research.

Whatever the statistics, these are our children. They show up at school, in our classrooms, and on our playgrounds, and they live with their caregivers within our communities. We are legally and, what is more, ethically required to help them. On a practical level, interventions that work will improve classroom and home life for everyone. This is where the Pyramid comes in.

Using the Pyramid means that we communicate a message of optimism and support. The "voice delivery," as described by one adolescent after he did not appreciate how the conversation went in one school where I observed the process, is a significant factor. *How* we say things, as any of us know from our own relationships, is as important as what we say. If this sounds obvious, just reflect on your own interactions and each person's tone of voice when one or more interactions did not go well. A fundamental aspect of communication is what our tone and nonverbal messages say. (The adage in speech therapy is that two-thirds of communication is nonverbal.) Again, we know this, but it often gets forgotten when a child is struggling and we are trying to regain control of a challenging situation—or when we are angry, or resentful, that this child who we have been invested in trying to help has been disruptive, angry, sarcastic, or outright aggressive.

The implication of control mastery theory is that, as much as possible, we are communicating that the Pyramid is a way to promote and maintain a child's safety. The moment it becomes, in the child's mind, a weapon of some sort, a way to try to exert control over the child, its ability to create safety is suspect. Even in the best of circumstances, it does not mean children are necessarily delighted to have such an instrument intruding into their lives. Nonetheless, safety emerges out of the support plan's structure, ongoing relationships, feedback, and built-in opportunities to both reflect and learn new coping strategies. In short, control mastery offers a theoretical foundation for why, as best we can, we should hang in there with these hurting children during their bleakest times.

When creating the Pyramid with any child, there is no one specific way to adapt the principles of CBT or the body-oriented models discussed above. This is not a manualized approach. Rather, both approaches lend themselves to what they do best: help hurting children question their understanding of the present and future despite what they may have experienced in the past. Or, if their trauma is ongoing, it allows them to separate out the safe aspects of their lives from those that are not. (Obviously, if there is active, enduring abuse, this needs to be reported right away.)

Understanding their physical sensations, those sudden alarms and pulses of anxiety that represent the body's holding of trauma, is integral to children's progress. All of this is incorporated into the Pyramid by having that very discussion, exploring how to use this knowledge in all three phases of prevention, redirection, and crisis intervention. One question I routinely ask is how children calm their body when upset, which leads the discussion from there. I have yet to meet a child who did not understand this question even if the child struggles to recognize when the change in internal state has taken place. How do children know they are upset? What tells them?

Similarly, children may understand the question even when they have no clue about possible solutions.

It is similar with CBT. The Pyramid is built around the idea that children's thoughts, especially when they are triggered, may lead them to misunderstand social cues and messages. We go to great lengths to communicate the idea that children are not necessarily wrong in their conclusions, only that they need to stop and investigate before acting. We look at strategies for how to accomplish this, such as slowing their breathing and rate of thoughts—these are examples of moving into Kahneman's System 2 thinking. We also want to help them consider what questions to ask. This is individual to every child, but the process has its own pattern. Learning new skills in the realm of what psychologists typically refer to as "reality testing" is a critical step. How do children know that someone is angry and rejecting of them? How do they know they are not safe? Which cues are they reading that lead to those conclusions? Do these same conclusions seem to fit a pattern of how the child makes assumptions? My favorite questions are in the realm of a basic "How do you know this?" and "Is there another way to understand it?" These kinds of questions should be incorporated into any problem-solving discussion when using the Pyramid. And these questions only work if the child feels comfortable enough with who it is that is asking; otherwise they shut down the dialogue.

While it may sound as though its introduction is lengthy, the Pyramid generally can be presented and discussed in approximately 20 minutes, with further review as needed. Children often have questions once they have first sat with the model. In some instances, there are repeated queries about why it is needed in the first place. I prefer a planned follow-up, a shorter one, prior to starting the intervention, especially because many children need time to think about their objections, questions, and any additional input they want to offer.

If at the center of it, therapy is about developing new meaning, the Pyramid is a seamless fit. Its purpose as a support plan is to generate the continual sense that help is available, but at the same time it promotes an underlying message of self-agency, growth, and capability. This is how new meaning making happens; it is the result of interactions that offer a different tenor and some hope for trust to build. Children may test the theory to see if the safety and support are real. In reality, they usually do test it. This is where our willingness to stay with it is most urgent. The predictability of the plan, based on the child's input as well as the adults', strengthens the notion that trust can take root. One child told me a few weeks into using it that this was the first time she had "faith" in adults, a comment that had real significance given her history of abuse and long periods of neglect.

Thus it is not only about the technical aspects of using the Pyramid. We need to think carefully about how we present it, how we will actively listen to the child's feedback (and perhaps a related torrent of resentment), and how we will continue to communicate around its use. These are not therapy moments, but they involve many of the same qualities of good therapy: openness, caring, a willingness to listen and sit with a child's pain, and, yes, compassion. Progress will not come in a straight line, nor should we expect this.

Promoting Resilience and Post-Traumatic Growth

Every one of the therapy models discussed earlier in the chapter, no matter what it emphasizes clinically and how it is implemented, should at its center promote resilience and post-traumatic growth. With so much ongoing talk about trauma and PTSD, it is critical to note that children, even those who have experienced some of the worst traumas, can continue to thrive in spite of what they have faced. As one 13-year-old girl told me, "[The traumatic episode] happened to me, it was really horrible, but it doesn't explain who I am as a person." Her statement reflects advanced wisdom for a child so young, but she had been through a lifetime of hardship and worked remarkably hard to reach a healthier—and frankly, much happier—place in her life. Hers was, among other things, a successful, long-term foster care placement that contributed to making this possible.

The idea of post-traumatic growth grew out of the work of two psychologists, Tedeschi and Calhoun, during the mid-1990s. Looking to ancient religious and philosophical beliefs about suffering, they found that people not only overcome trauma but can also adopt new meaning about the value and beauty of life (Tedeschi & Calhoun, 1995). They offer the noteworthy distinction that *resilience* reflects the idea of returning to a previous level of functioning, whereas *post-traumatic growth* suggests an even higher level of growth.

Later theorists, such as Rendon (2016), continued researching and promoting the discussion of post-traumatic growth. Parallel to this movement was the work of Seligman (and other psychologists), who developed positive psychology in 1998, a therapeutic perspective that remains very much in use today. Much of this thinking, especially at first, focused on adult development, but it is clearly applicable to children as well. In short, positive psychology emphasizes health and well-being rather than what is wrong or dysfunctional in people's lives. Consistent with what happens when there are competing theories in psychology, an active debate has emerged over the real-life benefits of implementing this model. Nonetheless, I find little argument in helping children see and accept their strengths. One way of understanding this approach is that it can provide a kind of therapeutic blueprint for working toward post-traumatic growth. If this sounds simple, it is critical to remember that children with trauma often struggle mightily with this process.

Equally important to the idea of promoting hope, we have to be careful not to communicate that we *expect* growth in any particular way. It is easy to slip into this stance. And we certainly need to avoid coming across as though we demand it. In our zeal and genuine good intentions to let hurting children know that life can improve, that we want them to feel better, we can unwittingly pressure them and leave them feeling worse. They are not necessarily supposed to "get over it." I have spoken with children who bitterly complain that "we don't get it" or that, in essence, we are not sensitive to their suffering. One child told me that the push to "heal" had everything to do with her surviving parent's guilt and nothing to do with her. Another child said he felt "ambushed" every time someone pressured him to talk about how he can "move on." Trying to press for change or to set the bar too high—no matter one's role in relation to the child—is an understandable but virtually never successful overreaction. It is a delicate balancing act, to promote hope and at the same time avoid pushing too hard, but one we must reflect on and continually monitor. Even though sitting with, and sometimes having to absorb, a child's pain is demanding, our relationship and ability to help are contingent on how well we are able to maintain that balance.

What, then, might post-traumatic growth look like in a child with PTSD? For me, and for many of the clinicians I asked, it comes down to reaching a new level of self-compassion. Self-compassion is a form of openness represented by greater caring and self-acceptance, a transformation from the intense and often relentless self-blame—and shame—that can consume these children. It may be (and often is) accompanied by an increased sense of empathy and awareness of others; in ideal situations, you can witness a wider perspective appear in front of your eyes. It is a privilege to watch such a process unfold. In addition, children often seem less anxious, less self-absorbed, and more able to take smart risks. Behaviorally, over time, you tend to see fewer major outbursts and shut downs, and, notably, recovery times, when they do occur, are faster. One child told me he handles frustration better and does not "break down" every time he cannot figure out something or faces disappointment.

Post-traumatic growth is a goal but not always a reality for every child, and it happens along a continuum. Again, if a child can learn some concrete bounce-back skills—resilience—it may be as much progress as the child can make at that time. But I have witnessed such growth often enough to know that it does occur, which is what other clinicians report as well. If nothing else, we should aim for such an outcome but without pressure, a sense of negative judgment, or a message of outright blame when it does not. Progress is jagged, even in the most positive scenarios. As much as possible, we should anticipate this reality.

That said, post-traumatic growth and positive psychology both offer the crucial reminder that children can survive their traumatic experiences and flourish. Not every child, surely, but many can. These ideas are a beacon of hope in what can be slow, difficult work, whether one is a clinician, teacher, school administrator, or caregiver. They encourage us to stay the course with children who shut down, run away, or become enraged. Which is exactly what these children need from us the most, especially when they have descended into the worst of their struggles.

The Pyramid furnishes a forum for all of this. It recognizes the complexity of grief and childhood behavior. It offers us a platform from which to plan and work, just as it does for these children. Ultimately, it contributes to the specific nature of our conversations and shapes what we need to provide. Referring to it as a support plan encompasses all this and makes explicit what the process is set up to do. At its best, the Pyramid provides the space, structure, caring, and attention to support the most traumatized children.

CHAPTER NINE

Two Students

Speaking of Esther

The following case study is based on parts of an exchange I had with a teacher. She agreed with my request to include it here, but details about the student have been carefully altered. The case is therefore a composite and not attributable to any specific child.

Background information: Esther is a 14-year-old, 8th-grade girl attending a rural elementary school that is primarily white. (She repeated 2nd grade due to many absences the year before.) She describes herself as a "Black girl" although I came to discover that she is biracial, a fact she has chosen to hide from her teachers and peers. Her father, for whom she seems to have a deep well of bitterness, is also biracial. Her mother identifies as a person of color. Esther moved into this district three years ago, after her family was filed on with the Department of Children and Families in another state. After two previous short-term stints in foster care and one longer-term stay with her grandmother, Esther has lived with one or both parents. (Her father has been in and out of the house, based first on substance abuse and then on a three-year jail sentence also related to drugs.) She has older half-siblings on both her mother's and father's side, but she has little relationship with any of them and considers herself an only child.

When she is under stress, Esther becomes increasingly disorganized in her thinking, emotions, and problem-solving skills. This shows up even in how she speaks; her stories suddenly take wide tangents without circling back to their original points. Sometimes an underlay of bitterness and anger erupts, seemingly out of nowhere. None of this is intentional; it represents the churning she describes using various terms for feeling overwhelmed. Her primary teacher during the school day, Ms. Avery, says that she can be a joy one-to-one but is sometimes a "real challenge" during group activities. In these situations, Esther talks over other students, gets frustrated if someone does not understand or agree with her point of view, and can become loud and somewhat combative. She needs to be right. Her agitation is just below the surface if not directly out in the open during these times.

At the same time, Esther is funny, sensitive, loving toward animals and immensely kind to other children she perceives as getting what she calls "the short end of the stick." Esther is wonderful with younger children. While she often struggles with traditional academic subjects, she is strong in art, music, and athletics. And she is an exceptionally talented singer, a role in which she seems most self-assured and at ease.

Ms. Avery is white and middle-aged, something the two of them had to navigate during the beginning of the school year. Esther said she "figured" her new teacher would be racially insensitive but then came to comprehend things differently as the school year progressed. Still, her behavioral problems have only increased. This includes blurting out, defiance, lying, and some verbal aggression toward other girls in her grade. Esther also says that people are "yelling" at her even when others in the room perceive only typical conversational volume and no evidence of anything in the way of overt hostility directed to her. Whether there are more subtle factors, microaggressions, that contribute to other students making her uncomfortable or putting her on the defensive is unknown, but none have been witnessed by adults in the school.

Esther was diagnosed at an early age with PTSD, ADHD, and ODD. The latter two labels came first, which is not entirely surprising since they are often in place before a child's trauma is recognized. Based on those labels, she was viewed purely as an externalizer. I was surprised not to see anxiety added to that list given her presentation; historically (and still today), she is described as "fluttering" around the classroom, and she often seems startled if not unnerved by anything unexpected happening around her. Medications for ADHD made her "crazy"—she hated how she felt during the various medication trials—and these were finally discontinued by her grandmother. Her later diagnosis of PTSD was based on a number of factors, not the least of which was sexual abuse by her father's brother who lived with them at one point. This was not a single event but one that went on for almost a full year until Esther finally told someone in her neighborhood. Her uncle was imprisoned as a result, worsening Esther's stress because, in essence, her father blamed her for this outcome.

When Esther breaks down behaviorally in school, she becomes argumentative and sometimes belligerent. Or, as she refers to it, things "get my back up." There does not appear to be a specific pattern as to when this occurs, although any struggle with an academic task is a frequent precursor (or what behaviorists refer to as an "antecedent"). Classroom interruptions are common. When she lies, her stories are typically about making herself, in her eyes, look better in front of her peers; she chronicles tales of family wealth and trips to exotic places in what clearly seems an attempt to impress others and feel more connected. But, as often happens in such situations, it usually leads to other students pulling away from her because they recognize that these stores are untrue.

It is this array of behaviors that underlies my back-and-forth sessions with Ms. Avery, who expresses confusion, sadness, and equal parts frustration and worry over Esther's behavior. She knows Esther has had a tough, unsettled upbringing, but she is not aware of many of the distressing details. A significant aspect of her disappointment is about wanting strongly to help this child and feeling badly that she has made what seems to her so little in the way of progress.

As Ms. Avery put it, "I'm really not sure how to help her. And I find myself getting more and more frustrated with her, especially since I know and she knows she's not telling the truth when she tells those stories. She disrupts the class every day, and sometimes I'm relieved if she's absent. It makes me feel really bad to say that, but the disruptions and arguments are hard to deal with. Honestly, I'm at a loss."

While these words are more honest and transparent than many educators might be willing to acknowledge, numerous teachers have students whose behavior they struggle to make sense of. What is more, they become distressed over how to help such students. I find that, perhaps paradoxically, it is the *most* competent teachers—those who regularly develop strong relationships with their students and establish clear, predictable guidelines in their classrooms—who find it the most troubling when they cannot figure out consistent ways to provide support. This makes sense, since their commitment and their usual methods of reaching students are typically successful. As we know, children with PTSD often bring a unique kind of challenge, one that stretches beyond our usual ways of making connections.

For Ms. Avery, Esther was a new test of skills, even though she had been teaching for many years and, to put it succinctly, excelled both in teaching academic skills and interacting with children (and thus "managing behavior"). For one thing, Esther did not trust closeness; she had felt close to the uncle who ultimately abused her and, as a result, this walled her off from virtually any adult who attempted to form a relationship with her. Yet, somehow, she inched her way toward Ms. Avery but not without many fits and starts. One day, after quietly being asked not to interrupt the class, she told Ms. Avery—not in front of other students, however—that she "hated her." And she stood there and glared at her. It was after this event that a very upset Ms. Avery reached out for help.

Our initial step was to talk about trauma and the components of PTSD but not the specifics of Esther's history; I do not share those unless a child and guardian consent to it and the information is critically relevant to what the teacher is seeing in the classroom. I explained (as I typically do) that the child has a history of trauma and loss and what this can mean in terms of the following: behavior, relational style, mood, attention, self-regulation, lying, coping skills, and social interactions—and academic output—and not only in isolation but the possible intersection among all of these factors.

Why offer a kind of psychoeducational first step when a teacher is desperately in need of some concrete repair strategies? The reason is that while Ms. Avery and many if not most other teachers have had some degree of professional development in trauma and how to create "trauma-informed" classrooms, most tell me that they do not feel at all confident or competent in this area. I find it important to normalize these statements since trauma-informed teaching is not yet a significant part of their training and not something they were historically expected to know. Nonetheless, I am always grateful to teachers willing to go out on a limb and learn more. There was, fortunately, no question about this when it came to Ms. Avery.

As our discussion progressed, I could see visible relief in Ms. Avery's face and posture. She had been blaming herself and thinking that she had "failed" this child. She began to grasp more fully why it might make sense for Esther to avoid getting too close to her too quickly, and why admonishing (or even trying to redirect) her publicly—in front of her peers—might lead to a self-protective outburst. She also began to more fully understand how this child could be so impulsive when stressed—and could thus blurt out in large-group activities—and why Esther's social relationships were shaky, if not volatile. And maybe most of all, she could understand why Esther was inconsistent in her work production and lied so frequently. None of this was sanctioned as acceptable behavior, but it explained a great deal of what Ms. Avery and other teachers were observing. It also set the stage for us to develop subsequent steps.

Next was for Ms. Avery to meet individually with Esther. She let Esther know that she wanted to "try some things differently" to see if these changes might be helpful. One such item was an agreement to avoid reprimanding her in front of classmates if at all possible. They set up a signal that Ms. Avery would use to let Esther know she was interrupting; the two of them also brainstormed ways for Esther to "wait," including scribbling down her ideas so they did not get lost. Ms. Avery went out of her way to quietly praise Esther every time she saw her begin to interrupt and then stop herself. This was a bright child, and she was perfectly aware that things were not going well. I could see from an outside vantage point how much Esther's attitude toward her teacher began gradually to soften, even if there were plenty of ups and downs. The wall of mistrust Esther built to protect herself—based on her history and experience—took time to even start to come down, but she clearly understood, at least intellectually, that her teacher was making every attempt to help her.

Why the school counselor was not already directly involved in working with Esther I had no idea, but I requested her participation. Esther could name but not reliably apply a single coping skill and had only a vague notion of what this might mean. When she was stressed at home, she either left the house to find some neighborhood kids, many of whom she did not like or get along with, or smoked marijuana on her own. Clearly, having the counselor's involvement seemed like an obvious need. What I learned later, however, is that this counselor had included Esther in a group, and it had gone disastrously; as a result, I think, she pulled away from Esther and offered no additional services. Having her back in the picture and ready to work individually once per week with Esther was a significant plus. For Esther, reviewing and practicing coping skills, including those for self-regulation, would be critical to progress. This made her time with the counselor a necessity, although they needed some extra time at first to build a working relationship.

With these aspects in place and Esther's mother in agreement—and, fortunately, Esther as well, which surprised almost everyone—we moved to developing a Pyramid. *How* the idea was presented to her was a critical factor. She was not initially warm to the notion of any kind of formal plan, but she came around when she understood that it was genuinely an attempt to help and, significantly, not something she could "fail." (As she put it, "I've screwed up way too many times. Not looking for more.") In the first section, *prevention*, we identified the need for Esther to be referred to an outside therapist. Similarly, we noted a request for her to see her primary care physician. By getting a signed release from her mother, we were able to ask the PCP to help advocate for outside therapy and to consider referring Esther for a medication evaluation. Other preventive steps involved her newly learned coping skills and building in time during the day for her to take breaks to practice them. As someone who intrinsically understood controlled breathing as a result of her many hours spent singing, she took almost immediately to these kinds of approaches. There are many—"Butterfly Breathing" and "Hot Chocolate Breathing" are two commonly used ones—but the point is that Esther gravitated to them.

Another preventive approach was to introduce Esther to the school resource officer (SRO). It was initially stressful for her, and at the last moment, she pleaded to avoid doing it, but it did not take long for her to connect with this woman, also a person of color and someone who exuded a calming presence. Having watched both of her parents get arrested by police officers—her father on more than a few occasions—she harbored a dread of them. Learning that Officer Grimes was available as a helping resource—a significant reframing of how she perceived the role of police—and as another person who could help her get calm if she became overwhelmed and escalated, was a relief to her.

An effective redirection for Esther was the wording "give and take," a prompt that school staff could use to remind her to step back and listen to someone else, whether an adult or a peer. Because Esther could become consumed by being in control, this phrase prompted her to step back if possible and wait a moment before speaking. She came up with these cue words herself, which certainly increased the likelihood that she would respond effectively. Rather than hearing them as a threat or demand, she slowly began to comprehend them as a message of help.

Esther typically did not escalate to the point of crisis in school. When this did occur, staff moved other students out of the room and allowed Esther the time and space to decompress. Because she had the capacity to come down on her own, this approach made sense. Some of the teachers resented the interruption, however, and expressed that it was disruptive to their teaching. Ms. Avery was open, as she said, to "whatever works." The nice news is that, as Esther built a repertoire of self-calming skills, she began to leave the room on her own when she became too escalated to maintain herself. The assistant principal set up a designated place for her to go and she would head straight there. Over the course of the year, this became increasingly unnecessary. She began to calm herself by staying *in* the presence of trusted adults rather than fleeing, an important aspect of her growth.

I do not mean to sugarcoat the story. There were many fits and starts, but overall, Esther made good progress. Her mood, academics, and social relationships all improved. She relied on the Pyramid as a sort of guide, and the feedback meetings were instrumental in helping clarify when she was beginning to, in her words, "go the wrong way." In school, we began to see a more cheerful child. The fact that her mother was stable during this time certainly contributed to her success, as did the advent of outside therapy. In addition, having a supportive teacher like Ms. Avery was undoubtedly instrumental to her progress.

Learning about Jake

Like our first case study, this is a composite story so that no one individual could be identified. Given the sensitivity of the content, this is critical.

Background information: Jake is white, almost 11, and in 5th grade. His is another story of a traumatic upbringing. He was sexually abused by his father, a man with an extensive drug and alcohol history, over the course of some unknown number of years when he was younger; this was before his mother discovered what was happening and filed a police report. The father is no longer in his life, a fact that brings him feelings of both great relief and abject guilt.

Jake was diagnosed with PTSD, anxiety, and depression early in 4th grade, when he first began to see a therapist. He was also evaluated in school, where it was discovered that his processing speed, despite average intelligence, scored only in the fifth percentile. In observing this boy, the realities of shame become readily apparent; he tries to disappear in almost every way imaginable. It is almost as if he is able to make himself smaller. He would wrap himself in a hoodie so that his face was barely visible. Since wearing hoodies has been banned in school, he has used a blanket whenever he can get his hands on one. He has been found in cubbies and other hidden-away spots in school and sometimes ducks under his desk in the classroom. Jake chooses to sit alone at lunch; when he is asked to join the other students, it is as if he is physically present but somehow located in another universe. Jake avoids classroom tasks, does not participate verbally, takes constant breaks in the back of the room, and will sometimes run away if asked to rejoin the group. The word *avoidance* comes instantly to mind when observing him. According to one of his teachers, Mr. Jefferson, who teaches English and social studies, Jake looks like he would "rather be anywhere else. If he could, he would just become invisible."

Jake is not at all mean or aggressive toward other people, but there is a reported history of self-harm. He has cut himself with a razor in hard-to-see places, such as his upper thighs and arms, on a number of occasions. Other students seem to sense that "something is wrong" and for the most part they leave him alone. The fact that he is a good athlete earns him credibility, especially among the boys, which seems to protect him from getting teased or put down. He looks sad and distant, sometimes even "vacant"; his teachers worry about him. As a result, he has been allowed to take breaks whenever he needs or wants them. His grades are poor except in math, a subject in which he has consistently done well.

Jake's outside therapist was not in touch with the school, something the school counselor tried hard to rectify, which, given Jake's complex history, made good sense. Not only did the school need to know what the outside therapist was trying to teach him skill-wise but the school counselor, Ms. Golic, was firm in her belief that the mother was not an accurate reporter of Jake's status. She commented on the mother's "huge guilt" and attempts to hold onto the idea that he was "doing fine." This is understandable given the context, but the therapist needs an accurate portrayal of Jake's functioning if she is to offer meaningful help.

For teachers, it was important to learn about both complex trauma and slow processing speed in more detail (not the details of his abuse, however, even though some asked). Since Jake tested at the fifth percentile for processing, he is frequently—as he says—"completely lost" in classes. Perhaps this is why he does better in math, because the math curriculum his school uses, a flipped classroom approach, is based more on active learning during class time and less on listening tasks. At home, Jake listens repeat-edly to the online lectures. He wants to do well and becomes frustrated when he does not. His other academic classes are taught in a more tradi-tional way, making him anxious that he is falling behind and, in his words, "stupid." As noted, this is very common among children with slow cogni-tive processing.

For Jake, this frightening sense of not doing well enough is compounded by the experience of his father telling him he was a "loser," a "dumb kid," and a "momma's boy." Apparently, this derision was frequent, and Jake continues to hold those hurtful statements in mind. Falling behind in classes reinforces these negative beliefs. He becomes more shut down, leading to his disap-pearances, sometimes right in the classroom when he puts himself under his desk.

In presenting the idea of the Pyramid, Ms. Golic asked Jake which teach-ers he wanted to join the two of them for the initial discussion. He named only Mr. Simpson, his math teacher and someone with whom he felt more comfortable than any other educator in the building. Mr. Simpson, a gentle, easygoing man with three children of his own, was happy to participate in the conversation.

What Jake wanted to know first was what would happen when he would "disappear" from, or within, the room. In other words, he asked for the crisis intervention plan first. He understood that others were concerned about this behavior and indicated that it bothered him as well. He found it confusing and upsetting, especially because he recognized that other children would find it different, if not, in his wording, "weird."

The Pyramid incorporated many different interventions, some of which Jake was able to suggest indirectly or at least agree to when they were pro-posed. Having a solid relationship with both adults in the room no doubt contributed to making the process go smoothly. It was explicitly framed as a brainstorming and problem-solving time; no opening was left for him to infer that he "screwed up." Ms. Golic was sensitive to the fact that Jake would instantly perceive the session as a negative reflection of him, as he was attuned to do, unless she quickly conveyed a competing, positive message.

Preventive steps included requesting the school psychologist to describe processing speed and his outside therapist to clearly explain PTSD to Jake; he was surprisingly eager to know more. Ms. Golic followed up by having a similar conversation with him in school. Understanding why he suddenly found himself on the move when under stress was a significant relief. We also asked the therapist to help him identify and label his negative emotions (the NED we discussed in an earlier chapter) so that he could begin to develop better strategies for handling them. In school, Ms. Golic followed up by using some DBT-related strategies in the attempt to help him learn to tolerate emotional distress. Jake enjoyed writing—not a common occurrence when someone has both trauma and slow processing speed. He started using a journal to record his negative thoughts and to both reframe and link them to coping responses.

As noted, the teachers were offered professional development specific to slow cognitive processing, which supported them in modifying their approaches to delivering instruction in the classroom. For example, Mr. Jefferson and Jake developed an agreement in which Jake would do his best to listen to the initial instructions and Mr. Jefferson would quietly follow up by checking in with him for understanding. This goes back to our earlier discussion about ensuring that students know we are here to help them avoid failure; Jake desperately needed this kind of lifeline. When he understood and could believe that the repeated instructions had nothing to do with being "stupid" and everything to do with the neurological reality of slow processing, he accepted help without complaint. These are simple interventions, but putting them into a clear, integrated format for Jake—and for everyone involved with him—made a significant difference.

Redirection was important to helping Jake. His tendency had been to disappear in full and then react negatively to people's attempts to reach him. A simple strategy was for staff to note, when he began to present as shut down, that he might "need some help." Other students did not pick up on this all that much because offering assistance was a common refrain in school. But Jake knew from discussions and follow-up meetings about the Pyramid what this meant. He knew that he needed to do his best to "step out of it" and reengage. Sometimes this meant going to the quiet corner for two minutes, breathing deeply and looking at a book, and then returning. He wanted to be with the class and doing what everyone else was doing, so task avoidance was not a concern. Teachers made a point of reinforcing him with a gentle nod—he did not want anything more than this—every time he left and then returned on his own.

As Jake began to develop new coping skills for managing distress, there was a gradual decline in the number of times he would suddenly disappear. He seemed, according to one of his teachers, less "vacant" and more engaged. Notably, it took less time for him to recover from an incident. When he did reach the crisis intervention stage, the adults around him spoke in a quiet tone, only one person talking at any moment, so that he could begin to reorient rather than flee even more intensely. The trust he established with his teachers and counselor played an integral role in his progress; he said, "[I] finally believe that they are on my side."

Jake had a couple of moderately significant incidents going forward, but he made great improvement overall. The Pyramid was a way to organize and clarify steps, both for him and for school staff. His mother adapted it to use at home, because Jake tended to have similar disappearances at home. The Pyramid provided a blueprint, a systematizing structure, and language, made necessary by adults' anxiety when he would, without warning, leave physically or, moreover, mentally. It is stressful for any of us to manage in these moments; one staff person joked—maybe only half-joked—that the Pyramid was as much for them as it was for Jake. This is not a unique observation when the Pyramid works effectively as an intervention.

Conclusions and Final Thoughts

The goal of this book has been to conduct a thoughtful look at what it means for a child to have trauma. The Pyramid is derived from that understanding. If it is to improve methodologically as a helping tool, a critical next step is to design outcome research for studying the Pyramid in detail. While I have seen significant progress in many cases, a systematic, large-scale investigation is needed. Such data should help us determine ways to refine the Pyramid going into the future and build on what works. It is, in short, an ongoing and evolving process.

It is also an enormously necessary one. A sobering study by Maynard, Farina, Dell, and Kelly (2019, p. 1) finds the following: "Despite growing support and increased rate of which trauma-informed approaches are being promoted and implemented in schools, evidence to support this approach is lacking." Much work remains to be done, with well-designed research a crucial component of this.

In addition, we should be mindful of an important study from the Jefferson Education Exchange (Jacobson, 2019) showing that only 16% of teachers use research that might alter how they practice in the classroom. If this is true overall, even relating to instructional methods, the percentage is likely lower when it comes to interventions geared to helping emotionally and behaviorally challenged children with PTSD. The study also found that educators prefer research that is presented in practical ways and fits with the "contexts" in which they work. These findings should guide how we offer professional development and other forms of adult support.

In the introduction to this book, Diana Fosha identifies the distressing sense of "unbearable aloneness." It has been a theme of this book, to recognize that children with PTSD—beyond the label—are hurting. While feelings of aloneness may be an expected part of human suffering, they can be an especially harsh intruder in traumatized children's sense of who they are and how they belong. This, ultimately, is what we need to try to help them confront. The Pyramid is one instrument for doing so, but the mission is vastly larger for all of us.

Abused children are victims. But sustaining a victim mindset is not necessarily helpful. It is in truth a delicate balance. We want to fully acknowledge and validate children's experiences, and their pain, but by continually referencing victimhood, we may be unwittingly contributing to their reliance on avoidance and their sense of powerlessness. Learning new coping skills—more effective ways to, in essence, live in community with others and with themselves—is a distinctly real possibility. Communicating that worldview can promote optimism and hope. We cannot rush the process, but embracing this central message is critical. The purpose of the Pyramid is to show any struggling child the possibility of going beyond the place of living as a victim—and, in a positive sense, the possibility of exerting some control over the process.

To implement and maintain such an intervention, there need to be community support and enough attention given to educator and caregiver self-care to be meaningful. These are critical needs for anyone to be able to engage in the often grueling work of relationship-building with severely traumatized children. This is not a matter of personal *weakness* or *failure*, words I hear too many times from adults in various roles. Maintaining our composure, our commitment, and even our willingness is not to be taken as a given. Too often, teachers and caregivers are expected to be compassionate without others recognizing how much is demanded of them when a child has been out of control, angry, or disruptive. This does not diminish the necessity. It speaks only to the idea that caregiving can be a thankless task, with many downs as well as ups, and it benefits everyone if the necessary support is offered. This has nothing to do with weakness and everything to do with being human.

Children do not operate in a vacuum. If we apply biopsychosocial thinking, it means that all of the contributors in a child's environment will affect how the child performs and feels. This returns us to Siegel's theory of *interpersonal neurology*. If a teacher has a trauma history, sometimes referred to as "teaching with trauma," it may be more difficult for the teacher to self-regulate emotionally during heated situations and help the child self-regulate. This is not blame; it recognizes that all of us function in a larger context that influences our capacity to manage our own emotions. It is no different for caregivers, whether parents, grandparents, or any other guardians, who bring their own experiences and perceptions to their interactions with children. If adults are highly stressed—and we know the overall levels are elevated for teachers—it means there is less anchoring (or the *co-regulation* we discussed earlier) available for children on the edge. Recognizing this, and building in the right kinds of supports, will help all of us.

In fact, this growing awareness of both child and adult stress in schools has led Kaiser Permanente and two other organizations to confront the issue directly (Berg, 2019). Called Resilience in School Environments, or RISE, the program targets school staff in implementing stress management strategies. By addressing stress in this way, the expectation is that children will benefit as a result. The Pyramid has a similar function in that it helps adults reduce stress by providing a clearly defined, organized, and predictable approach to use even in the worst of times. In other words, the model was created to benefit children with trauma as well as the adults who teach, counsel, and raise them—thus the rationale for referring to it as a "support plan."

Gale-force winds are pushing education toward more personalized learning approaches. There is a glaring recognition that simply using more of the same teaching methodology is not a road to a better future for all students. Funds are pouring into artificial-intelligence programs that will enhance how we build and implement these personalized learning models. We should take a similarly creative approach to teaching children with trauma. One-size-fits-all social-emotional programs will help many children but not those with the most severe trauma histories. Traditional behavior plans are generally unsuccessful in supporting progress, especially for those children who lack the necessary self-regulation skills. Carefully individualizing our approach to these children, through a structured and, at the same time, thoughtful and child-centered intervention, will allow us to take the next steps forward in helping them. Children who have suffered so much deserve nothing less.

References

Introduction

Ablon, J. S. (2018). *Change-able: How collaborative problem solving changes lives at home, at school, and at work.* New York, NY: TarcherPerigee.

Fosha, D. (2003). Dyadic regulation & experiential work with emotion & relatedness in trauma & disordered attachment. In M. F. Solomon & D. J. Siegel (Eds.), *Healing trauma: Attachment, trauma, the brain and the mind* (pp. 221–281). New York, NY: Norton.

Jennings, P. A. (2019). *The trauma-sensitive classroom: Building resilience with compassionate teaching.* New York, NY: Norton.

Lifton, R. J. (2017). *The Nazi doctors: Medical killing and the psychology of genocide.* New York, NY: Basic Books.

Regel, S., & Joseph, S. (2017). *Post-traumatic stress* (2nd ed.). New York, NY: Oxford University Press.

Chapter 1

Ainsworth, M. D. S. (1978). *Patterns of attachment: A psychological study of the strange situation.* Hillsdale, NJ: Lawrence Erlbaum Associates.

Brown, D. (2015, December). *Meditation in everyday living.* Conference proceedings. Boston, MA.

Collaborative for Academic, Social and Emotional Learning (CASEL). (2019). Core SEL competencies. Retrieved from https://casel.org/core-compete ncies/

Davies, W. (2018). *Nervous states: Democracy and the decline of reason.* New York, NY: Norton.

Fischer, R. (2015, January 20). Failure to launch syndrome: What does it mean to launch successfully? *Psychology Today.* Retrieved from https://www

.psychologytoday.com/us/blog/failure-launch/201501/failure-launch
-syndrome

Fisher, J. (2017). *Healing the fragmented selves of trauma survivors: Overcoming internal self-alienation.* New York, NY: Routledge.

Jones, E. J., Lam, P. H., Hoffer, L. C., Chen, E., & Schreier, H. M. C. (2018). Chronic stress and adolescent health: The moderating role of emotion regulation. *Psychosomatic Medicine, 80*(8), 764–773.

Levine, J. E. (2007). *Learning from behavior: How to understand and help challenging children in school.* Westport, CT: Praeger.

Levine, P. A., & Kline, M. (2006). *Trauma through a child's eyes: Awakening the ordinary miracle of healing.* Berkeley, CA: North Atlantic Books.

Mandler, G. (2012). Mind-pops: Psychologists begin to study an unusual form of Proustian memory. *Scientific American, 307*(2), 28.

National Child Traumatic Stress Network. (2019). Trauma types. Retrieved from https://www.nctsn.org/what-is-child-trauma/trauma-types

Perry, B. D. (2007). *Stress, trauma and post-traumatic stress disorders in children.* London, England: Jessica Kingsley Publishers.

Richmond, R. L. (2018). *Boundaries: Protecting yourself from emotional harm.* Seattle, WA: Amazon Services.

Rowe, M. B. (1986). Wait time: Slowing down may be a way of speeding up! *Journal of Teacher Education, 37*(1), 43–50.

Saxe, G. N., Van der Kolk, B. A., Berkowitz, R., Chinman, G., Hall, K., Lieberg, G., & Schwartz, J. (1993). Dissociative disorders in psychiatric inpatients. *American Journal of Psychiatry, 150*(7), 1037–1042.

Siegel, D. J. (2012). *The developing mind.* New York, NY: Guilford Press.

Solms, M. (2019, October 19). *Consciousness affect and learning: Unconscious, defense and therapy.* Keynote presented at the meeting of the Neuropsychoanalysis Association, New York, NY.

Sorrels, B. (2015). *Reaching and teaching children exposed to trauma.* Boston, MA: Gryphon House.

Stanford Children's Health. (2019). Posttraumatic stress disorder (PTSD) in children. Retrieved from https://www.stanfordchildrens.org/en/topic/default ?id=posttraumatic-stress-disorder-ptsd-in-children-90-P02579

Starr, L. R., Hershenberg, R., Shaw, Z. A., Li, Y. I., & Santee, A. C. (2019). The perils of murky emotions: Emotion differentiation moderates the prospective relationship between naturalistic stress exposure and adolescent depression. *Emotion.* Advance online publication. https://doi.org/10.1037 /emo0000630

Teater, B. (2014). Case study 2-1: Social work practice from an ecological perspective. In C. W. LeCroy (Ed.), *Case studies in social work practice* (3rd ed., pp. 35–44). Belmont, CA: Brooks/Cole.

Thomas, A., & Chess, S. (1977). *Temperament and development.* New York, NY: Brunner/Mazel.

Westover, T. (2018). *Educated: A memoir.* New York, NY: Random House.

Chapter 2

Bhengu, M. J. (2014, April 23). The spiritual significance of the Egyptian pyramids [Web log post]. Retrieved from https://jbhengu.wordpress.com/2014/04/23/the-spiritual-significance-of-the-great-pyramids-of-egypt/

Bryan, B. (Producer), Nash, N. (Producer), & Villena, F. (Director). (2019). *Any One of Us*. Mexico: Red Bull Films.

Comas-Díaz, L. (2016). Racial trauma recovery: A race-informed therapeutic approach to racial wounds. In A. N. Alvarez, C. T. H. Liang, & H. A. Neville (Eds.), *The cost of racism for people of color: Contextualizing experiences of discrimination* (pp. 249–272). Washington, DC: American Psychological Association.

Copeland, W. E., Shanahan, L., Hinesley, J. Chan, R. F., Aberg, K. A., Fairbank, J. A., . . . Costello, E. J. (2018). Association of childhood trauma exposure with adult psychiatric disorders and functional outcomes. *JAMA Network Open, 1*(7), e184493.

Curtin, S. C., & Heron, M. (2019). Death rates due to suicide and homicide among persons aged 10–24: United States, 2000–2017. NCHS Data Brief, no. 352. Hyattsville, MD: National Center for Health Statistics.

DeRubeis, L., Kim, K. H. S., Ardalan, F., Tanis, T., Galynker, I., & Cohen, L. (2016, May, 14–18). *The relationship between childhood trauma, impulsivity, and suicidality in an inpatient sample* [Poster presentation]. 2016 Annual Meeting of the American Psychiatric Association, Atlanta, GA. Young Investigators' New Research 1–017.

Duncan, B. L., Miller, S. D., Wampold, B. E., & Hubble, M. A. (Eds.). (2010). *The heart & soul of change: Delivering what works in therapy* (2nd ed.). Washington, DC: American Psychological Association.

Gershenson, S., Hart, C., Hyman, J., Lindsay, C., & Papageorge, N. W. (2018). *The long-run impacts of same-race teachers* (NBER Working Paper 25254). National Bureau of Economic Research, Inc.

Hall, P., & Simeral, A. (2008). *Building teachers' capacity for success: A collaborative approach for coaches and school leaders*. Alexandria, VA: Association for Supervision and Curriculum Development (ASCD).

Kahneman, D. (2011). *Thinking, fast and slow*. New York, NY: Farrar, Straus and Giroux.

Kuypers, L. M. (2011). *Zones of regulation: A curriculum designed to foster self-regulation and emotional control*. Santa Clara, CA: Think Social Publishing.

Levine, J. E. (2007). *Learning from behavior: How to understand and help challenging children in school*. Westport, CT: Praeger.

MacDonald, D. K. (2016). Crisis theory and types of crisis [post]. Retrieved from http://dustinkmacdonald.com/crisis-theory-types-crisis/

Maynard, B. R., Solis, M. R., Miller, V. L., & Brendel, K. E. (2017). Mindfulness-based interventions for improving cognition, academic achievement, behavior, and socioemotional functioning of primary and secondary school students. *Campbell Systematic Reviews, 13*(1), 1–144.

National Child Traumatic Stress Network, Justice Consortium, Schools Committee, and Culture Consortium. (2017). *Addressing race and trauma in the classroom: A resource for educators.* Los Angeles, CA, and Durham, NC: National Center for Child Traumatic Stress.

O'Brien, B. S., & Sher, L. (2013). Child sexual abuse and the pathophysiology of suicide in adolescents and adults. *International Journal of Adolescent Mental Health, 25*(3), 201–205.

Ratey, J. J., & Manning, R. (2014). *Go wild: Free your body and mind from the afflictions of civilization.* Boston, MA: Little, Brown and Company.

Santoro, D. A. (2018). *Demoralized: Why teachers leave the profession they love and how they can stay.* Cambridge, MA: Harvard University Press.

Schön, D. A. (1983). *The reflective practitioner: How professionals think in action.* New York, NY: Basic Books.

Sparks, S. D. (2019, August 20). Brain images used to tease out how top teachers connect with students. *Education Week.*

U.S. Census Bureau. (2017). *National survey of children's behavior.* Washington, DC: U.S. Census Bureau.

Van der Kolk, B. A. (2014). *The body keeps the score: Brain, mind, and body in the healing of trauma.* New York, NY: Viking.

Chapter 3

Johnson, S. (Producer). (2019, February 19). The science of empathy: What researchers want teachers to know [Audio podcast]. EdSurge Podcast. Retrieved from https://www.edsurge.com/news/2019-02-19-the-science -of-empathy-what-researchers-want-teachers-to-know

Miller, W. R., & Rollnick, S. (2013). *Motivational interviewing: Helping people change* (3rd ed.). New York, NY: Guilford Press.

Norcross, J. C., & Wampold, B. E. (2019). Evidence-based psychotherapy responsiveness: The third task force. In J. C. Norcross & B. E. Wampold (Eds.), *Psychotherapy relationships that work. Volume 2: Evidence-based therapist responsiveness* (3rd ed., pp. 1–15). New York, NY: Oxford University Press.

Riess, H. (2017). The science of empathy. *Journal of Patient Experience, 4*(2), 74–77.

Shea, Shawn C. (2017). *Psychiatric interviewing: The art of understanding: A Practical Guide for Psychiatrists, Psychologists, Counselors, Social Workers, Nurses, and Other Mental Health Professionals* (3rd ed.). London, England: Elsevier.

Chapter 4

Bradshaw, J. (2005). *Healing the shame that binds you* (2nd ed.). Deerfield Beach, FL: Health Communications.

Burgo, J. (2018). *Shame: Free yourself, find joy, and build true self-esteem*. New York, NY: St. Martin's Essentials.

Coles, R. (2000). *The moral life of children*. Boston, MA: Atlantic Monthly Press.

Fisher, J. (2017). *Healing the fragmented selves of trauma survivors*. London, England: Routledge.

Hallward, A. (2014, December 8). *How telling our silenced stories can change the world*. TEDx Talk.

Hyde, L. (2019). *A primer for forgetting: Getting past the past*. New York, NY: Farrar, Straus and Giroux.

Kelly, V. C., & Lamia, M. C. (2018). *The upside of shame*. New York, NY: Norton.

Piaget, J. (1936). *Origins of intelligence in the child*. London, England: Routledge & Kegan Paul.

Van der Kolk, B. A. (2014). *The body keeps the score: Brain, mind, and body in the healing of trauma*. New York, NY: Viking.

Winnicott, D. W. (1960). The theory of the parent-infant relationship. *International Journal of Psychoanalysis, 41*, 585–595.

Chapter 5

Ariely, D. (2012). *The (honest) truth about dishonesty: How we lie to everyone—especially ourselves*. New York, NY: HarperCollins.

Bok, S. (1999). *Lying: Moral choice in public and private life*. New York, NY: Vintage Books.

Bronson, P., & Merryman, A. (2009). *NurtureShock: New thinking about children*. New York, NY: Twelve Publishing.

Ekman, P. (1987). *Why kids lie: How parents can encourage truthfulness*. New York, NY: Penguin Books.

Ford, C., King, B. H., & Hollender, M. (1988). Lies and liars: Psychiatric aspects of prevarication. *American Journal of Psychiatry, 145*(5), 554–562.

Harris, S. (2013). *Lying*. Opelousas, LA: Four Elephants Press.

Levine, J. E. (2007). *Learning from behavior: How to understand and help challenging children in school*. Westport, CT: Praeger.

Chapter 6

Augustine, C. H., Engberg, G. E., Grimm, G. E., Lee, E., Wang, E. L, Christianson, K., & Joseph, A. A. (2018). *Can restorative practices improve school climate and curb suspensions? An evaluation of the impact of restorative practices in a mid-sized urban school district*. Santa Monica, CA: Rand Corporation.

Engel, B. (2013, July 2013). How compassion can heal shame from childhood. *Psychology Today*.

Fronius, T., Persson, H., Guckenburg, S., Hurley, N., & Petrosino, A. (2019). *Restorative justice in schools: An updated research review*. San Francisco, CA: WestEd Justice & Prevention Training Center.

Kohn, A. (1993). *Punished by rewards: The trouble with gold stars, incentive plans, A's, praise, and other bribes.* New York, NY: Houghton Mifflin.

Virues-Ortega, J. (2006). The case against B. F. Skinner 45 years later: An encounter with N. Chomsky. *Journal of Behavior Analysis, 29*(2), 243–251.

Wachtel, T. (2016). *Defining restorative.* Bethlehem, PA: International Institute for Restorative Practices.

Chapter 7

Kegan, R. (1994). *In over our heads: The mental demands of modern life.* Cambridge, MA: Harvard University Press.

Pearlman, S. J. (2014). Meaning making and making meaning meaningful: The relationship between language and thought in critical pedagogy. *International Journal of Critical Pedagogy, 5*(2), 100–113.

Zittoun, T., & Brinkmann, S. (2012). Learning as meaning making. In N. M. Seel (Ed.), *Encyclopedia of the sciences of learning* (pp. 1809–1811). Boston, MA: Springer.

Chapter 8

Cohen, J. A., & Mannarino, A. P. (2008). Trauma-focused cognitive behavioural therapy for children and parents. *Journal of Child and Adolescent Mental Health, 13*(4), 158–162.

Dana, D. (2019, March/April). The touch taboo. *Psychotherapy Networker.*

David, D., Cristea, I., & Hofmann, S. G. (2018). Why cognitive behavioral therapy is the current gold standard of psychotherapy. *Frontiers in Psychiatry, 9*(4). https://doi.org/10.3389/fpsyt.2018.00004.

Davies, W. (2018). *Nervous states: Democracy and the decline of reason.* New York, NY: Norton.

Fosha, D. (2000). *The transforming power of affect: A model for accelerated change.* New York, NY: Basic Books.

Ghandour, R. M., Sherman, L. J., Vladutiu, C. J., Ali, M. M., Lynch, S. E., Bitsko, R. H., & Blumberg, S. J. (2019, March). Prevalence and treatment of depression, anxiety, and conduct problems in U.S. children. *Journal of Pediatrics, 206,* 256–267.e3.

Ginwright, S. (2018, May 31). The future of healing: Shifting from trauma informed care to healing centered engagement. *Medium.*

Jennings, P. A. (2019). *The trauma-sensitive classroom: Building resilience with compassionate teaching.* New York, NY: Norton.

Kahneman, D. (2011). *Thinking, fast and slow.* New York, NY: Farrar, Straus and Giroux.

Levine, P. A. (2010). *In an unspoken voice: How the body releases trauma and restores goodness.* Berkeley, CA: North Atlantic Books.

Mahler, K. J. (2016). Interoception: *The eighth sensory system: Practical solutions for improving self-regulation, self-awareness and social understanding of individuals with autism spectrum and related disorders.* Shawnee, KS: AAPC Publishing.

Mazza, J. J., Dexter-Mazza, E. T., Miller, A. L., Rathus, J. H. and Murphy, H. E. (2016). *DBT skills in schools: Skills training for emotional problem solving for adolescents (DBT STEPS-A).* New York, NY: Guilford Press.

Perry, B. D., & Szalavitz, M. (2017). *The boy who was raised as a dog.* NY: Basic Books.

Presidential Task Force on Posttraumatic Stress Disorder and Trauma in Children and Adolescents. (2008). Children and trauma: Update for mental health professionals. Washington, DC: Presidential Task Force on Posttraumatic Stress Disorder and Trauma in Children and Adolescents. Retrieved from https://www.apa.org/pi/families/resources/children-trauma-update

Rendon, J. (2016). *Upside: The new science of posttraumatic growth.* New York, NY: Touchstone.

Rotaru, T. S., & Rusu, A. (2016). A meta-analysis for the efficacy of hypnotherapy in alleviating PTSD symptoms. *International Journal of Clinical and Experimental Hypnosis, 64*(1), 116–36.

Siegel, D. J. (2012). *The pocket guide to interpersonal neurobiology: An integrative handbook of the mind.* New York, NY: Norton.

Siegel, D. J., & Bryson, T. P. (2011). *The whole-brain child: 12 revolutionary strategies to nurture your child's developing mind.* New York, NY: Delacorte Press.

Tedeschi, R. G., & Calhoun, L. G. (1995). *Trauma and transformation: Growing in the aftermath of suffering.* Thousand Oaks, CA: Sage Publications.

Van der Kolk, B. A. (2014). *The body keeps the score: Brain, mind, and body in the healing of trauma.* New York, NY: Viking.

Weiss, J., & Sampson, H. (1986). *The psychoanalytic process: Theory, clinical observation, & empirical research.* New York, NY: Guilford Press.

Conclusions and Final Thoughts

Berg, J. (2019, December 15). Kaiser plans to use virtual and in-person resources to target stress, anxiety in schools. *MedCity News.*

Jacobson, L. (2019, November 21). Survey: Most educators find research hard to access. *Education Dive.*

Maynard, B. R., Farina, A., Dell, N. A., & Kelly, M. S. (2019). Effects of trauma-informed approaches in schools: A systematic review. *Campbell Systematic Reviews, 15*(1–2), e1018.

Index

Note: Page numbers followed by *f* indicate figures.

About the Author

James E. Levine, PhD, LICSW, began working in schools in 1980 before starting graduate school in social work, which led to a master's degree and then, some years of clinical practice later, a PhD from Simmons College (now University), in Boston. He has been a licensed clinician since 1987. Much of his work has focused on the intersection of trauma, mental health, developmental skills, and behavior. This emphasis led to starting an organization that, to this day, combines consultation to schools and public agencies across New England, outpatient psychotherapy, and comprehensive psychological evaluations. This work includes risk assessments and, when needed, the creation of support plans. His previous book, *Learning from Behavior*, was published in 2007, first in hardcover, then in paperback, and, later, in an international edition. Dr. Levine has presented across the United States on various topics relating to children's mental health and behavior.